Advance Praise for *Body Odyssey*

"An insightful and intriguing work."

Richard J. Leider, Founder of The Inventure Group, and best-selling author of
The Power of Purpose, Repacking Your Bags, and
Claiming Your Place at the Fire

"Body Odyssey beautifully unveils the creative promise of aging. It's an important book, worth studying and discussing for its provocative wisdom, worth savoring for its dramatic, honest storytelling."

Susan Perlstein, executive director,
National Center for Creative Aging and Elders Share the Arts

"I loved it! It made me think about my body in a whole new way. I'll be buying copies to give to my friends."

Jan Hively, senior advisor, Vital Aging Network

"*Body Odyssey* brings to life the passion—the fire—of aging in a beautiful and thought-provoking manner. Samples, in telling the story of her own 'Body Odyssey,' awakened me to the stories carried in my body."

Barbara Ginsberg, Ed.D., My Turn director,
Kingsborough Community College, CUNY

"Pat Samples is an astute, sensitive, and resolutely honest recorder of the lessons our bodies have to teach us if we will but heed them."

Lawrence Sutin, professor, MFA Writing Program, Hamline University

"Samples spontaneously sings and dances her emotional and spiritual stories, letting her body take the lead. She shows us ritual turning points, letting stories of hurt and happiness be revealed as the body is given freedom of expression to let the dance begin."

Andrea Sherman, Ph.D., project director,
Consortium of New York Geriatric Education Centers in New York City

D1593313

"Our bodies can be beautifully expressive at all ages, and *Body Odyssey* offers stunning close-ups of their wisdom and creativity. Samples magically captures the language of movement on the page in a most engaging way."

Manfred Fischbeck, artistic director, Group Motion Dance Company

"This writing is engaged and vital, possessing an urgency and passion that keep me reading. I trust what this voice tells me about how to work and live in the body and find myself repeatedly attracted to the way of living described on these pages."

Barrie Jean Borich, author of My Lesbian Husband:
Landscapes of a Marriage, *and writing professor*

"This is not only a riveting book to read, but one to savor in memory long after. Even in the midst of her most significant trauma, a kidnapping, Samples shows unusual grace and ultimate forgiveness."

Margot Fortunato Galt, author of The Story in History: Writing Your Way
into the American Experience, *and writing professor*

"Pat Samples' stories of courageously facing the challenges of graceful aging will be an inspiration to many women on the same journey."

Lavinia Plonka, author of What Are You Afraid Of?

"Inspiring, soulful, practical—a 'must-have' for anyone who has a body! Samples deciphers the meaning of her own bodily discomforts, faces old demons, and shows us, through her own rich life stories, how to learn from the body's wisdom. She helps to free us from the dread of aging."

Deborah Antinori, drama therapist and licensed professional counselor

Body Odyssey

Lessons from the Bones and Belly

Michele,
Enjoy your
body odyssey!
Pat Temple

Other books by Pat Samples

Daily Comforts for Caregivers

Self-Care for Caregivers: A Twelve Step Approach
(Pat Samples, Diane & Marvin Larsen)

Comfort and Be Comforted: Reflections for Caregivers

With Open Arms (Gene Sylvestre and Pat Samples)

The Twelve Steps and Dual Disorders
(Tim Hamilton and Pat Samples)

The Twelve Steps and Dual Disorders Workbook
(Tim Hamilton and Pat Samples)

Older Adults in Treatment

Older Adults after Treatment

Portions of this book are adapted
from articles that have appeared in

The Phoenix

A View from the Loft

Body Odyssey

LESSONS

from

THE BONES

and

BELLY

Pat Samples

SYREN BOOK COMPANY
Minneapolis

Most Syren Books are available at special quantity discounts for
bulk purchases for sales promotions, premiums, fund-raising,
and educational needs. For details, write

Syren Book Company
Special Sales Department
5120 Cedar Lake Road
Minneapolis, MN 55416

Published by
Syren Book Company
5120 Cedar Lake Road
Minneapolis, MN 55416

Printed in the United States of America on acid-free paper

ISBN-13: 978-0-929636-51-1
ISBN-10: 0-929636-51-1

LCCN 2005930341

Cover design by Kyle G. Hunter
Book design by Wendy Holdman

To order additional copies of this book see the form
at the back of this book or go to www.itascabooks.com

Contents

Acknowledgments

Splendid teachers have introduced me to the wisdom of our bodies. I am grateful especially to Karen Roeper, Manfred Fischbeck, Cherie McCoy, and Ron Petit.

Thanks to the members of the improvisational movement group I lead each week, who have allowed me to develop new ways to explore and delight in the body's creativity. Every week, dancing with them takes me to a state of awe.

I owe a great debt to Thomas Wright, co-creator of the Writing Your Own Permission Slip course, from which many of the book's examples are drawn.

Many artists and advocates with a passion for vital and creative aging have inspired my own work in aging and particularly the writing of this book. Among those whose leadership and personal encouragement have been a lighthouse for me are Susan Perlstein, Sally Hebson, Jan Hively, Jane Cunningham, Connie Goldman, Evelyn Fairbanks, and Maria Genné. I also give credit to authors Meridel Le Sueur, Brenda Ueland, James Hillman, and Sam Keen, whose writings and example awakened my excitement about writing and about aging with vigor.

Members of the faculty in Hamline University's Master of Fine Arts in Writing program nursed me through the writing of this book with great competence and care. I especially thank the members of my thesis committee, Margot Galt, Larry Sutin, and Barrie Jean Borich.

My writing group stayed with me through the development of the book, believed in it, and gave me critical, practical feedback. Audrey Rogness, Carol Nulsen, Lisa Deitz, Marie

Michael, and Linda Varvel contributed much insight to this manuscript.

Tim McIndoo brought to the editing of this book his exquisite sensitivity as he nudged me toward clarity and simplicity in my writing. Thank you, Tim. I also want to acknowledge Sid Farrar for his valuable guidance about publishing.

Friends make all the difference. They teach me, encourage me, challenge me, and love me. Thank you for helping me shape and hold on to my dreams: Rita Mays, Anne Boever, Marjorie Spagl, Ron Nelsen, Kathy Olson, Linda Gearke, Cindy Gray, Barb Grohs, Joy Anderson, Julia Jergensen-Edelman, Larry Freeborg, Jeff Sylvestre, Cynthia Ryden, Brian Brooks, Tracy Leverentz, Michael Leverentz, and Dennis Verrett. Thanks also to my son, André Samples, for his loving support and faith in me.

Preface

$\mathcal{Y}$our body has stories to tell. So does mine. Our sad, fearful, surprising, and joyful moments register in tightened muscles, quickened heartbeat, a rush of energy. These somatic imprints stay with us, especially if they are often repeated, holding in our bodies our lifetime of experience. Our bodies become home to our stories. The longer we live, the more stories await our discovery.

Body Odyssey: Lessons from the Bones and Belly is an invitation to get to know our bodies in a new way so we can harvest these stories. Because our bodies are archives of our experience, we can turn to them as a generous resource for wisdom, creativity, and learning, especially in our older years. In these pages, I illustrate a mindful approach to discovering what they can reveal through stories of my own body's revelations. I also draw on the wisdom and experiences of others. My hope is that through reading these stories and reflections, you will be intrigued by the mysteries of your own body.

But most important, this book calls for a change in how we regard the aging body. In much of American culture, the bodies of the old have too long been the subject of despair and ridicule. In the recent push for "healthy aging," older bodies have become the object of anti-aging toning and tucking campaigns. But what if our bodies were regarded as treasure chests, filled with an abundance of hidden riches that can nourish, heal, and energize us until our last breath? What if we were willing to learn from them? What if we could creatively express the stories they hold through writing, dancing, or other artistic forms?

As I have raised these questions in classes, talks, and workshops across the United States, people have expressed surprise and delight at the hidden jewels they find when they befriend their bodies in this new way. I wanted many more people to have this experience. That's why I wrote this book. I've even included an appendix that suggests specific activities to help you expand your own body awareness. I've also listed resources, including information about body-based therapies and teachings that might assist you in your discovery process. Should some of the stories and exercises in this book stir up deeply disturbing memories held in your body, professional guidance may be especially important for you in order to gain the wisdom and healing that are possible from listening to your body.

I came to understand the aging body's amazing gifts through an eclectic course of study that began when I turned fifty. I wanted to know how to make the most of the second half of my life, and since my body was giving me many signals of distress, I found myself curious to learn from its messages. Body awareness teachers and healers helped me awaken to the sources of my pain and to unexpressed vitality. I learned from mindfulness practices what my body wanted and what it was capable of, moment by moment. I participated in improvisational dance and theatre activities. I learned how to stop and rest. Little by little, I came to notice and cherish my somatic wisdom and creativity.

At the same time, as an author and speaker on family caregiving, I had become markedly aware of physical frailty and its impact on family members and friends. I saw caregivers too often wearing out and dying faster than the people they cared for. I couldn't help but wonder if there were lessons to learn from these bodies as they were failing.

I have devoted the past decade not only to pursuing my personal body odyssey but to expanding my understanding of how all of us, especially as we age, can become more conscious and appreciative of what our bodies have to offer. I decided to pursue a master's degree in human development, with an emphasis on conscious aging and the body, which involved a great deal of self-designed fieldwork. I observed, interviewed, read, and wrote. But my main course of study in the past decade has been with somatic and spiritual teachers, artists, fellow professionals in the aging field, older people who have touched my life, and other friends and acquaintances who have chosen to live with conscious awareness and intention in their bodies. My ultimate teacher, of course, has been my body, and this learning continues day by day.

Since we learn best what we teach, I have been teaching and speaking on the wisdom of our aging bodies for much of the past decade. Again and again, I am thrilled by the opportunity to be a witness as people come to discover, write, sing, dance, celebrate—and sometimes revise—the stories their bodies tell them. Teaching about aging and the body also helps me stay attentive to my own body's emerging stories. Let me begin *Body Odyssey* by telling you a story that my body told me one day, taking me quite by surprise.

Part One

Don't Bury Me Before I Die

—⟶—

What is going on when our bodies cry out?
Maybe they have lived too long without anyone hearing their stories.

🌀 Chapter One

When Terror Wants to Have Its Say

*T*en of us sit on floor cushions around workshop leader Cherie McCoy. We are here in this home in an old St. Paul neighborhood to discover how attention to our bodies can help heal wounds of the psyche.

I am excited, curious, nervous. Nearly fifty years old, I've attended plenty of classes and workshops on personal development, yet I'm on edge. I don't know quite what to expect from this Self Acceptance Training. I'm only here because I trust my friend who recommended I attend. As I wait for the workshop to begin, I'm aware of gnawing body troubles—back pain, shoulder tension, tight jaw—plus a collection of anxieties and fears. Nothing life-threatening, but often life-diminishing. They're the reason I'm here. After having tried many ways to solve these problems, I hope Cherie can help me figure out what's got me stuck. Yet, I question whether I should be here. Will I like these people? Will I be asked to do something weird? How will I manage to sit on the floor for two days?

Cherie's size and smile remind me of a cherub. As she gets the workshop under way, she welcomes us in a voice as soothing as a kitten's purr. She asks us to keep what we hear in the workshop confidential. Then she tells us that each person will get an hour or more of personal help from her in front of the group. First, though, we'll each have about ten minutes to introduce ourselves and explain why we're here.

One by one, stories of trouble unfold. An older woman tells of a strained relationship with her daughter. A mid-twenties man wants to figure out his calling. A balding, heavyset man is tired of feeling depressed. And so it goes around the circle. With each person, Cherie points out where the story rests in the person's body.

Hannah*, a tall, stiff-necked young woman, wants to be more accepting of her chronic pain. Cherie smiles maternally and says, "Hannah, check in with your body and see if you can feel where you carry the resistance to the pain."

"I have this lump in my throat a lot of the time. It's hard to swallow."

"Is there something you're having trouble swallowing?" Cherie asks tenderly, as if taking the woman into her arms.

Hannah starts to choke. "I've been swallowing my fear. I've been trying so hard to be brave." The choking changes to sobbing. "I don't know how long I can do this. The pain is so wearing."

"Yes, the pain is wearing, and so is holding in all of the resistance to the pain—trying so hard to be brave. Let the tears come that want to come, and let all the fear be there."

"It feels huge."

"Yes. It is huge. That's why you have a lump in your throat. Your fear is big and it wants to have a voice. It's choking you to get your attention."

Hannah's face softens into a smile. The tears stop, she sits up straighter.

"I've been trying to be so positive, to visualize health, to stay strong."

"You can be positive and strong and brave, and still feel the fear."

Hannah takes a big breath and nods.

---

* Some names and details in this book have been changed to protect the privacy of the people described and to simplify the storytelling.

"Is there anything else for now?"

"No."

"We can do more with this later, if you want, Hannah."

"Thanks."

One by one over the next ninety minutes, the others in the circle introduce their stories and Cherie guides them through their troubled terrain. I am both stunned and entranced by how quickly she works with them to unravel the emotional tangles. By the time the person next to me makes her introduction, I'm barely listening. Instead I'm puzzling about how Cherie does this. Unlike other workshop leaders I've met, Cherie is not offering formulas for success or tips for overcoming obstacles. Rather, she unveils and welcomes obstacles as teachers. People seem to be shifting remarkably fast from pain to relief and even to acceptance. What's happening seems strange, eerie, yet intriguing.

I realize it will be my turn soon; I grow increasingly nervous. I have no idea what I'll say. Before coming, I had hoped to get some help with the panic attacks I had been experiencing for a number of years, but they seem too scary to mention now. I feel as if my story will fall apart if I try to tell it; as if I will fall apart.

Bam! A noise explodes behind me. I jump a half-inch off of my cushion, my hands fly in the air, and my head whirls around to see the source of the disturbance. A metal folding chair has fallen to the floor. My whole body begins to shudder.

As my neighbor continues with her introduction, I try to stop my jittery moves, so as not to be distracting, to politely wait my turn, to avoid being noticed. But the trembling intensifies. Confusion, shame, fear, and heat envelope me.

After my neighbor finishes, there is silence. Cherie turns her soft eyes toward me. The whole group is watching. My eyes dart about; my gaze drops to the floor. I know my voice will tremble if I try to speak. I don't know what's happening to me or what to say.

Cherie speaks. "It looks like there might be something going on with you, Pat."

I try to make my jaw work. All I can do is shudder and nod.

"Would you like to talk about it?" She pauses. "You don't have to if you don't want to."

Somehow Cherie's permission not to speak allows me to do so, though my lips barely part: "I just got scared when that chair fell over," I say, as if that would explain my obvious terror.

"What was it about that chair falling that was so frightening?"

"I don't know. I can't figure out why it's bothering me so much. I can't stop shaking." The palsied tremors embarrass me.

"It's okay for you to be shaking here. We can try to find out what the shaking is about, if that's all right with you."

I nod, though I feel unsure.

"Did it remind you of something?"

My father lies in a coffin. I am eight and I am curious to see the bullet hole in his forehead. But it's not there.

The man gets in behind the wheel of my car and pushes me over to the passenger's side. It is dark, yet I see a glint of light on the gun pointing toward me.

"It sounded like a gunshot," I say.

"Do you have some memory of a gunshot?"

"Well, not of a gunshot really. But two memories of guns came to mind when the chair fell. Maybe it has something to do with one of those." The possibility seems very far-fetched.

"What were they?" Cherie's tone of voice is permissive, offering an invitation I know I can decline safely. But I respond because I don't know what else to do. Mostly my thoughts race, garbled. I am trying to will my shaking to stop; it won't. I am half curled over as I speak, trying to disappear.

"One was my father shooting himself when I was a kid. I didn't see that actually happen, but when I think of a gun, that's what I think of. There was also the gun that was pointed at me when I was kidnapped and held hostage a few years ago."

Within the first few minutes of my turn, I have spilled out into this group of strangers the two worst nightmares of my life. Something about Cherie's presence, her voice, her kindness hints at a distant open gate in the tortuous prison that encamps me. I trust her—but only barely—to get me out safely, to stop the terror. At the moment, she seems like my only hope. I desperately need to trust someone.

"Which of these incidents with guns do you think this is about?"

"The kidnapping."

"Would you like to work on that?" Cherie's inviting smile offers the same assurance I've just seen open the way for others in the group.

"I don't know if I have any choice," I say, succumbing to her tender solicitation with a voice still shaky but tinged with laughter. It's a relief to drop the self-control that has failed to hide my untidy feelings and make light of my strange behaviors.

As the others have done, I move over and sit directly in front of Cherie.

"Tell us what happened," she says, and after a long exhale, settles back to listen.

Drowsy after a long evening's work, I yawn deeply as I drive into the alley behind my house in a northern section of Minneapolis. Moments later, I park my red station wagon in the dark garage, scoop up my tote bag, and swing open the car door, eager to head inside the house and get under the covers. I skip the usual cautious glance into the rearview mirror to make sure I'm alone before getting out.

The glance would have been too late anyway. As I turn to place my feet on the garage floor, a large figure in a long black coat lunges at me. I am jolted wide awake. Unclear words come at me from a male voice. I am terrified. I think, *Rape!* I draw back and raise my feet to fend him off, yelling, "No! No!"

"Be quiet or I'll shoot you!" he demands. Only now do I see a piece of shiny black metal pointing my way. I get quiet quickly.

"I just want a ride to Brooklyn Center," he announces firmly, yet with a tone of reassurance. I *am* reassured. Brooklyn Center is a nearby suburb, maybe ten minutes away. If that's all he wants, I can handle that. Mainly to calm myself, I put the keys back in the ignition and try to reassure him. "Okay, just get in," I say, "and I'll take you to Brooklyn Center." But he's not interested in my offer.

"Just get over. *Get over!*" He pushes his way into the driver's seat.

I hurriedly move as far over as I can, trembling as I press myself against the door on the passenger's side.

"Give me the keys."

I'm shaking so badly that I can barely respond, but wanting to get this over with in a hurry, I search for a voice and words.

"I think they're in the ignition." It is too dark to see. I start to open my door so the light will come on and reveal where they are. But I'm stopped by his abruptly raised weapon and a barked order, "Don't try anything!" His sharp reaction is my first clue he is terrified, too. But I have no time to absorb it.

"Where are the lights?" The question is a demand. "Turn them on!" I recoil at the idea of reaching across him to pull out the light knob, but he insists. As my hand and arm extend, he doesn't touch me. I'm relieved. I can see now the keys are indeed in place.

Using his left hand to point the weapon toward me and his right hand to grasp the wheel, he eases the car out of the garage and into the alley. I struggle in the brief silence to clear up the massive disorientation I'm feeling. *If this turns into rape, what do I do?* Barely able to concentrate, I scan my memory for any tips I may have heard about how to handle rape, including moves I learned in a self-defense class ten years earlier. What little I remember seems irrelevant in a car with a gun so close.

I had spent the evening working with a friend on a writing project about the divine spark that lives in each person and how to rely on that for guidance in all matters. I had come away feeling spiritually uplifted and strong. Now, underneath the trembling, I resurrect that feeling and pray. *Dear God, I've never had to deal with rape before. I don't know how to handle this. Show me what to do. This is in your hands.* Despite the fierce trembling, I now know I'll be all right, no matter what happens.

"I just want a ride to Brooklyn Center," the man cuts into my thoughts. I want to believe him. I do believe him.

He seems unsure where to turn at the end of the alley, so I begin giving him directions, quietly, politely, wanting to keep him calm, wanting to calm myself. But he turns the opposite way. Obviously, this ride to "Brooklyn Center" is going to take some detours.

He begins questioning me.

"Are you married?"

"Yes."

"Where is your husband?"

"At home."

My answers are brief and truthful. It seems dangerous to give him the personal information he asks for, yet I'm not used to lying and I don't want to take any chances on getting tripped up.

"When is the last time you had sex?"

So this is how it's going to start. I push myself more tightly against the door, cowering and shaking like a cornered cub.

"I don't want to discuss that." I surprise myself by my boldness.

He surprises me. "Don't worry, I'm not going to rape you."

I want to believe him, but his questioning has alarmed me. Yet, temporarily relieved, I blurt out, "Thank you."

Until now, I've been afraid to look at him, but I realize I'll want to be able to identify him later. I start to turn my head his way.

"Look the other way," he snaps, raising his weapon again. In the dark garage, I had only gotten a glimpse of his dark brown face, stocking cap, long black coat. His voice sounds youthful, his accent Southern. He is forceful each time he issues an order but otherwise conversational and even sometimes polite.

"How much money you got?"

"I don't know. About twenty dollars."

"That all?"

"I think so. I'm not sure." It's true I'm not sure. If I turn out to be wrong, I don't want him to think I lied. He might get even more edgy with the gun. I'd better win his trust if I hope to get out of this alive.

We ride slowly down Fremont Avenue. There is little traffic at eleven o'clock at night. He tells me to take out my purse, then asks, "You don't have a gun in there, do you?" He sounds nervous, suspicious, but he makes no abrupt move this time and does not raise his voice. I realize for the first time that he is afraid of me. I wonder how I can reassure him and find a way to trust him at the same time—find some common ground. *Is he basically a good person despite what he's doing now? What if I'm honest, decent, caring—will he react the same way?* I'm looking desperately for that divine spark.

I count out twelve dollars.

"Are you sure that's all?" he asks more than once, but by now he seems almost sheepish about questioning my word. I show him there is a little change. I'm too nervous to count it.

There is silence as he continues driving. I am shaking, both from fear and from the cold of the wintry night. At last he pulls into a parking lot of an apartment building. He turns off the motor and the lights. *Will there be rape after all?*

"May I have the money now?" His politeness seems ironic, but strangely sincere.

I hand it to him, being careful not to touch him.

"Thank you." He adds, "Can you write me a check?"

I tighten up. Twelve dollars I can afford to lose, but a large sum would greatly strain my limited resources. I don't answer. He says nothing, starts the car, and drives out of the lot.

"I'm going to tell you what will happen if you try to tell the police anything about this," he says, "or if I hear that anybody comes around asking about this, if this even shows up in the paper. I know your car. I know your license number. I know where you live. I will come back and kill you. Even if they arrest me, they won't give me more than a fine and I'll be out right away and I'll come back and I'll *kill* you."

I know he's right. I know he could terrorize me for months or years. I'd never feel safe. The trembling intensifies.

"Now, I'm not a bad person," he says, trying to soften the effects of his threats. "I'm only asking for fifty dollars. I'm not like some guys who would ask for a hundred or two hundred dollars or everything you got. A lot of guys would rape you, too, but I'm not going to do that."

He pauses. "How much do you have in the bank?" I had just balanced my account earlier in the day and had more than six hundred dollars.

"About three hundred dollars, I think," I say. I'm lying. Something in me refuses to give him everything I have.

"Will fifty dollars hurt you very much?" he asks, sounding genuinely concerned. "I just need fifty dollars for some transportation, so I can get around town and get a job," he explains. He sounds like a boy, wanting me to think well of him so I'll help him out.

After more driving, he stops in another parking lot and asks me to write him a fifty-dollar check. My hands shake so badly from fear and from the cold that it takes several attempts to open my checkbook. I write in large jagged scribbles.

"What's your name?" I ask, wondering how to fill in the "Pay to . . ."

"Larry Washington," he says, after repeating the earlier threats if I report him. Then he asks me where there's a bank that's open so he can cash the check.

"I don't think there's a bank open at this hour." I am stunned by his naïveté.

He seems surprised. I tell him he can cash it the next day, but he's convinced I'll call the police before he can do so. I reassure him that I won't call. I just want to end this whole ordeal and go home. I'm ready to pay fifty dollars for that privilege, but he's not buying it.

I decide on another tactic. Byerly's, a supermarket just outside the neighborhood, usually cashes checks easily, so I suggest we go there. When we arrive, he stops the car in the middle of the store's large, almost empty parking lot. As he prepares himself to go inside, he orders me to stay in the car. He threatens me again. He knows my car, knows where I live. He will find me and kill me and my husband. I am convinced. Besides, I remember that my phone number is on the check. Yes, he certainly could make my life miserable for years to come. I don't see a ready way to escape. There is no place to run to. Nearby stores are closed for the night. Even if I dashed across the parking lot, I reason, he could see me through the store's large glass doors and come back out to chase me. I'm sure he or his bullet could reach me. The risk seems too high.

"You need to look as sharp as possible," I say. Despite the threats, despite my fears, there is something about this young man that has awakened a maternal caring in me. Maybe it's the way he seems just as scared as I am. Maybe it's his periodic politeness or his youth. Maybe I'm convinced that indeed the fifty dollars will be his ticket to finding a job and becoming a responsible citizen so he won't think he has to do this again. He has said several times that he's "never done this before." I'm suddenly aware of how dull-witted he is (after all, he actually revealed his name to me and knew little about such basics as when banks close) and how powerless he must feel that he has come to rely on a gun for basic survival. For my sake and for his, I want him to succeed in cashing the check. It will be my ticket home and his means to pursue a job. In my mind, I try to wish away the gun and the threats and imagine just giving him the money as a gift.

At this point, things become almost comical. It occurs to me that a late-night, check cashing request by a young black man in this suburban supermarket for mostly affluent whites might not be easily honored. So, I become his coach.

"Comb your hair so you look nice. Act friendly. Try to look like you're a very responsible, trustworthy person," I advise him, like I might prepare my own son for a job interview. Out of the corner of my eye, I can see him taking off his long black coat, straightening his cap and his clothes. We become a team now, out to accomplish a joint mission, each doing what we have to do to protect ourselves in the process. He walks toward the store entrance. I am too cold and shaky to even consider jumping out of the car. I turn to watch him, a thin young man trying to walk tall. *Where were the elders who should have shepherded this child into proper manhood?*

He comes back quickly, sounding despondent. "They won't cash second-party checks."

"I'll go in and cash a check," I offer. I want to get this over with. Besides, I'm a persistent person. When I start something, I want to finish it.

"You'd do that for me?" His voice conveys surprise, appreciation, and a renewed suspicion all at once. Then, "You going to try to call the police or something, aren't you?"

"No, I won't. I promise. I know you could get back at me and I don't want to take that chance. I just want to get this over with so I can go home. Besides, I'd like to help you out so you can get a job." At last I convince him I'm sincere. With little further dialogue, he lets me go into the store. He parks the car right outside the entrance and promises to watch me all the time I'm inside. I hurriedly go in, get the money, and head back toward the door. Trembling and scanning the store, afraid someone will notice, I nearly bump into the manager. I open my mouth to speak to him, but car lights beaming through the door change my mind and I keep moving.

My captor seems genuinely grateful for my efforts, though he questions me about whether I reported the situation while inside the store. After he drives off, he takes several odd turns onto side streets, checking to see if we're being followed. Yet I sense a growing ease between us. Our difficult but joint mission has been successful. Larry has his money, and at last I'm heading home.

On the way, he tells me about himself. He has come to Minneapolis very recently, planning to live with his aunt, but she has moved and he has been unable to find her. The little money he came with has all gone for rent. He has been looking for work, he says. Jobs for young unskilled black men are, I know, not easy to come by.

"I saw a 'Help wanted' sign today," I say. "Do you want to know where?" By now, I really want to help Larry. I know he'd be better off, and so would society, if he were working rather than committing robberies or doing prison time.

"You'd just come and check to see if I was working there and then send the police," he says. The tone of his voice is not accusatory. It sounds as if he wants to trust me but can't under the circumstances. I know I can't convince him otherwise.

Now he is following my directions to get me home. The

tension has thinned. After a moment of quiet, he asks, "You prejudiced?"

Caught off guard, I hesitate, expecting some new twist to the evening, depending on my response.

"It's okay, you can tell me. I won't hold it against you," he says, with a lightness in his voice. On the one hand, I believe him; on the other hand, I know my reply had better be good.

"Let me tell you a funny story about that," I say, recalling a long-past incident. The memory from my familiar world, strange as it is in the middle of this situation, is especially welcome.

"I was working with a group of kids, many of them black and some white. I had them loaded on a bus to take them on a trip," I begin.

"You a teacher?" Larry interrupts, interested now.

"No, I was working at an arts learning center at the—"

"I'm an artist!" Larry butts in eagerly. "I'm a real good artist."

"I worked with a lot of young guys like you," I jump back in, "helping them get art lessons and music lessons and theatre classes."

"You did? I like art. I'm good at it." He says this excitedly, like a proud child. "But, go on with your story," he begs.

I tell him that once, while taking a group of students on a bus trip to a concert, I had passed the time by counting the number of people on the bus—the number of black people and the number of white people—and I had counted myself among the black people. I laugh as I recall how silly I felt when I realized that, in my efforts to promote interracial harmony, I had gone overboard.

Larry laughs with me, clearly enjoying my story. We are nearing my house and I feel myself relax a bit more. Though I'm still shaking, I have gotten used to it after what has seemed like hours of captivity. In a moment, I'm thrown off again. Larry turns a corner and begins driving around the neighborhood rather than heading directly for the street where I live. He isn't explaining. The silence seems long, unnerving. Gingerly, I ask him about his artwork and tell him I have just started a watercolor class myself. He tells me he has been to art school and that he has "won a lot of awards" for his artwork. "I'm real good at art, and it's not like I'm going to waste that. I'm going to use it." Once again, he assures me, "I'm not a bad person. I'm going to get a job." I tell him, truthfully, "I believe you."

Gradually, I realize he is driving around because he can't figure out how to end all of this. If he leaves me and walks away from the car, he's afraid I'll immediately call the police. And he clearly has come to care enough about me that he doesn't want to hurt me. He has trapped himself and doesn't know how to get out.

"Are you going to be all right when you get back home?" he wants to know.

I dig deep for the answer. "Yes, I will. I have this belief that God will take care of me no matter what happens, and he'll take care of you, too, and everything is going to turn out all right." I believed this from the beginning; now I'm all the more sure of it.

"I wish you hadn't mentioned God. Now I feel bad." There is a long silence. Then, "I'll be just as glad as you when this is over."

Larry pulls over to the curb about a half mile from my house. We both sit there, quiet. After a few minutes, he turns off the ignition and pockets his weapon. There are no rules of etiquette for ending a robbery. He steps out, but I don't hear him moving away and the car door remains open. I'm getting colder and finally glance in his direction. He is standing by the car door, looking at me. Out of habit, I still don't look at his face.

"Thank you very much for helping me out," he says in a quiet voice that rings of sincerity and shame.

"You're welcome."

"I'm really sorry about all this," he adds and walks away.

⟶

I didn't report the incident to the police. I didn't want to risk living with the fear of his threatened reprisals for years to come. Besides, I reasoned, even if he were caught, which was unlikely since I wouldn't be able to offer the police much of a description, I couldn't identify him.

More important, I'd made a promise and I hadn't made it lightly—even if it was under duress. I had made it because Larry reminded me of those many boys who had come to me when I worked at the art center, boys whose life in the streets and whose legacy of racism had carved a nasty imprint, but who underneath had compassionate hearts, artistic promise, and playful spirits. I was angry and sad about what their legacy had done to them. They needed strong, caring mentors, not punishment, to help get them on track. They needed someone to believe in them. Like so many of the boys I had known, Larry clearly had no one to show him the way. Society had let him down, and so, apparently, had his family. Though what he had done to me was wrong and stupid, I hadn't been hurt. I had been shaken—I was still shaking—but I'd get over it. Putting him behind bars wouldn't fix anything. What would prison do but expose him to more criminal influences? He'd come out and do worse things. So my reasoning went.

But Larry made a mistake. He tried to cash the check I'd given him. The storekeeper was suspicious and called the phone number on the check. When my husband answered the call, he told the storekeeper what had happened. Larry was arrested soon afterward and I was called by the police. They asked me to go down to the station and make a statement. I went. I decided I wanted the whole story told. When I met with the arresting officer, he told me he'd coaxed a confession from Larry, telling him, "Larry, the lady who gave you the check said you didn't seem like a bad person, so why don't you tell the truth." Larry, only eighteen years old and a long way from home, broke down and cried. The officer agreed with me that Larry seemed naive, sincere, and remorseful, not at all like the usual mugger. He said Larry was very, very scared of going to jail.

In the week that followed, I pondered the many implications of this incident. On the one hand, I hadn't slept at all the night of the incident, and my body continued to tremble for several days afterward. Every time I drove into my garage, a wave of terror washed over me, and I had to look behind me over and over before I could step out of the car. And I was angry and distraught that my week's plans got severely disrupted in the aftermath of this event. But none of these effects seemed all that important. Overriding them were the exhilaration and gratitude I felt for being able to trust God's guidance throughout the ordeal. It seemed miraculous that I had maintained the conviction of a divine spark in myself and in Larry, despite the danger and the terror. The strength I found in this experience gave me a new, deep-seated invincibility.

My gratitude, invincibility, and continuing faith in the divine spark meant I had a mission to accomplish—to help right the wrongs that had set the stage for Larry's actions. I wanted this young man out of jail and getting the help he needed. I knew whatever actions I took would affect him forever; I wanted to make sure I took the right ones.

The story of a woman I once interviewed inspired me. She had met the woman who murdered her son, forgiven her, and helped her when she got out of prison. Could I find a similar strain of heroism in myself? Could I try to get the charges dropped? Could I even work with Larry personally to help him get a job? After all, I had years of experience helping troubled young people.

But I couldn't go that far. I came to realize that not only did I have to regain my emotional equilibrium, I also had a troubled marriage to deal with, a son to parent, and other personal and business affairs needing my attention. I did talk to both the prosecuting and defense attorneys, however, and pleaded that they find a way to get Larry some job counseling and assistance rather than a prison sentence. I expected the massive and impersonal criminal justice system to dismiss me as naive, yet my intervention brought results. Instead of a state prison sentence, Larry got workhouse time and a long probation during which job placement would be a priority. "If you had told us you wanted the book thrown at him, we would've done it differently," the prosecuting attorney told me. "This guy is getting what might be the biggest break of his life."

That's what I wanted, for Larry to get a break, to find out that someone believed in him, even when he was at his lowest. I was convinced this kind of treatment would make a difference for him. I also wanted to believe for myself that this incident could have some redeeming outcome to it—the kind only forgiveness can bring. So, I wrote him this letter:

Dear Larry,

I have been thinking of you often since we met a few weeks ago. First, I want you to know I was certainly terrified the night you held me hostage and took my money. I trembled severely for some time afterward and am still scared when I go into my garage or to other places where I could be in danger again. I even get jumpy in my own house when I hear anything unusual. The whole incident created a series of other problems for me as well. I'm angry, and I certainly hope you never put anyone through something like that again.

But I have many other feelings as well. For one thing, I am grateful for what I have learned, including who my friends are and how I handle myself under that kind of pressure. I am also concerned for you. Even under those horrible circumstances, I saw a good heart in you and the desire to do well. I saw that you believed in yourself. I believe in you too, Larry. You are a wonderful child of God, and you deserve a good life. I pray that, although this may be a discouraging time for you now, you will look deep within your soul to find forgiveness for yourself and to know the forgiveness of God as well. You certainly have mine. Please use the time you spend in jail to look further inside yourself to discover and celebrate all the good that is there. Because you have all that good, consider how you can use it to fulfill your dreams and to make a contribution in the world. Then check in to job training and placement programs that will get you started on your way. I hope someday to hear how the way you handle this experience became the first step in proving how great you are.

A few weeks later, I received a neat, five-page handwritten reply on lined notebook paper. The letter contained repeated apologies and numerous expressions of gratitude. It spoke of Larry's regrets—"I felt bad about the situation. I didn't want to do it. I was tearful as I left your car." It included reassurances that "you don't have to worry about me hurting you." It even offered some friendly advice—"If someone approaches you whom you do not know, take precautions"—and a promise that "someday you *will* hear how this experience became the first step in proving how great I am."

At the end Larry added a postscript: "Thank you, I'm sorry, I love you, Mrs. Samples," accompanied by a smiley face drawing. On the next page was a four-stanza, crudely rhymed poem Larry had written, and following that, a drawing of a rose.

Sitting in the workshop on the pillow facing Cherie, these detailed memories of the kidnapping experience swamp my mind when she asks me to tell what happened. Barely able to talk, I relate aloud only a snapshot version of the story. My shaking body has already revealed its emotional essence. I finally speak because I am taken in by Cherie's rounded maternal form and face, her cushiony voice, and her warm eyes looking into mine.

"I drove into my garage late one evening and opened the car door, and this man came at me with a gun. I thought I was going to be raped, but he just wanted money. He drove me around for what seemed like hours."

I try to sound brave and in control, just reporting on what happened, as if from a distance, but I'm still shaking so fiercely the words come out in jerky segments.

"That must have been very scary." Cherie leans toward me, heart first.

"He was just a kid, just a young guy who hadn't figured out how to grow up. All he wanted was some money for bus fare so he could look for a job."

"But you were scared."

"Yes. But, I don't know why I'm shaking now. I wish this would stop. I really did okay at the time. I handled everything okay. I even tried to help him out afterward so he could get his life in better shape."

"I'm sure you did, but now your body is remembering the fear."

"But I was okay really. He didn't hurt me. In fact, he sent me a poem and a drawing from jail afterward."

"He kidnapped you. That's an awful thing to have happen to you."

"Yes, but . . ." My shuddering is now part shivering. I am growing cold. I can't think of what more to say.

"You were scared."

Her words sink in.

"Your body still remembers. I'm sure you did a beautiful job of handling the situation, but your body has never let go of the terror from the experience. Now it's ready. It wants to. It's remembering so it can let it go."

I don't understand exactly what she means, but I've had a glimpse of what she's done with the others in the group. I'm willing to find out what she suggests.

"So, what am I supposed to do?"

"You don't have to do anything. Your body is already doing it. You just get to let the feeling be there, and I'll be right here with you to help you go through it. I'll help make it safe for you to have all the terror you've been holding in all these years, so you don't have to hold on to it anymore."

"Okay." And then, feeling this has gone on way too long already, "But isn't my time about up?"

Cherie smiles. "We'll give you all the time you need."

She invites me to lie down on the carpet and covers me with an afghan. I curl up in a semifetal position, shuddering and shivering all the while and trying to stop. Cherie places her hands tenderly on my shoulder.

"Now, Pat, just go ahead and let the fear be there, the big fear that your body is telling you about. You don't have to do anything but let your body do what it's doing. Your body is very smart and it knows exactly what to do."

For what seems like an hour, my entire body shakes and flails as if prodded by an erratic, low-level electrical current. There is no holding back. The shuddering and shivering take over. At times the movements become jerky, a vibration striking my legs or my shoulders like lightning. The shaking feels like it will never stop. From time to time, Cherie's assuring voice encourages me, coaches me.

"It's hard work to carry around so much terror inside. Let it come out now. That's it. Yes."

She begins to name what happened to me that night long ago in a way I had never considered, or had dismissed back then.

"Your whole being was threatened. Your life was threatened. This must have been terrifying. It was an act of violence. Your right to safety was taken away. You lost your sense of security. What a scary, scary thing to have happen to you! Your body has been holding on to this terror all this time, all the memories of being so frightened. It wasn't safe to show them at the time. It wasn't safe to speak up and say no at the time. But, it's safe to do that now."

I am crying.

"Yes, let the tears come. The pain is very, very deep. It's ready to be healed. The tears are helping you heal. In our society, we aren't used to crying out loud, we aren't used to expressing our pain publicly. In other cultures, there is a lot of wailing. Here in this room all the sounds of our grief and our anger and our hurt can come out. It's all right to cry, to wail, to scream, to let out all the feelings that want to come out."

I start to sob. Waves of terror and racking grief take over. Sounds I have tried to stifle now come out in primal blurting eruptions.

"Your voice was shut down by having the gun pointing at you, but here there is no one to shut down your voice. So, Pat, you can say no here, you can tell this man who terrorized you to stop."

The tears and shaking subside a little as I consider her suggestion.

"No," I say weakly, wiping my eyes and nose of moisture. "No, don't do that." I feel foolish. He is not here now. But my body is shaking less.

"Why don't you sit up now so you can call up your full voice and say no."

I feel ready to sit up and I do.

"See if you let your voice match the power of the terror and the grief and the anger you're feeling. Let it be louder. Let your no be heard."

"No!" I am louder now.

"Good, Pat. Keep going. Louder."

"No! Stop that. Don't do that. Get away from me!" I'm not feeling foolish now.

"Good. Say, 'Get away from me' again, and let all the force of the terror you've been feeling back it up."

"Get away from me! Get away from me! Get . . . away . . . from . . . me! Stop it! Stop it! Stop it!"

"You have no right to do this," Cherie feeds me a line.

"You have no right to do this!" I am screaming now at the dark figure I remember. It is Larry, and it is not Larry. It is all the evil that moment came from and all that it created.

"I won't let you," Cherie offers another line.

"I won't let you. I . . . will . . . not . . . let . . . you. You will not do this to me. No! No! No! I hate it that you did this to me! I won't let you do it to me anymore! I won't let you."

My voice softens. I'm through yelling; now I've begun declaring with confidence. "I am free from you. I am free. You don't scare me."

I am now fully upright on my knees. My voice is clear. I am not shaking anymore. I take a very deep breath. The room is quiet. My whole body is throbbing, not with terror but with a pulsing sense of power. I barely notice the enormous exhaustion and achy residue of unbridled terror and tears.

Cherie smiles tenderly. "That was very courageous, Pat—very beautiful."

Now I feel tears of relief welling up. "Beautiful." This seems like a strange word, but like milk from the breast, I drink it in.

"I wish you could see your face. It's radiant. It's beautiful."

She offers, "Would you like me to hold you?" She widens her lap, and I collapse into her open arms. Once again I move into a semifetal position, but this time I am not afraid. I am home, safe. Cherie strokes my hair like an adoring mother, and rocks me gently.

🌀 Chapter Two

From Cover to Uncover

*I*t's been ten years since the long-lidded terror of being kidnapped rampaged through my body in Cherie McCoy's workshop, spurring my declaration of independence from this fright. Over those ten years, I have come to appreciate the body as a storyteller, teacher, and healer of the spirit. I have developed an avid interest in learning about the body's wisdom and power, and have shared my discoveries with others in my writings, speeches, classes, workshops, and other forums. My liberating interchange with Cherie was one of many experiences I've had—and witnessed—that demonstrate the wealth of revelation our bodies can offer us.

Our bodies are like storybooks, capable of illuminating in sentient detail our life experiences if we're willing to read them with fervent curiosity. During our lifetime, our eyes have catalogued billions of imprints of faces and places, some friendly, some not. Our ears have retained countless reverberations—of parental yells, school bells, and babies crying. We have recorded our history through sight, hearing, smell, touch, and taste, and also through our sense of balance, movement, spatial awareness, and intuitive knowing. Our pelvis remembers riding sleds and romping with lovers until sated, registering conclusions about safety and the transience of exhilaration. Our arms and torso know from experience the location and width of the bathroom doorway in our home even in pitch darkness. We "know" when a situation is dangerous and we pick up "good vibes" from people, in large part because we sense something familiar to our past experience. The more years we've lived, the larger these libraries of our lives grow, every experience imprinted in our bones and organs and sinew.

As children, we relied on our bodies as learning resources. Touching, tasting, and shaking things were our principal study habits. We also mimicked what interested us. Our bodies made a permanent register of these encounters and enactments, beginning to construct the archives from which we have since drawn. Running with flapping arms, trying to fly, we came to *know* our weight as heavier than the robin's in a way no book or schoolteacher could explain.

In much of Western culture, well-meaning adults insist all too soon that we learn to restrain our bodies. *Keep your eyes on the board. Be quiet and listen to what I tell you. Keep your hands to yourself. Walk in a straight line.* Twelve years or more of formal education restrict our body's engagement mainly to the use of our eyes and ears, hands and mouth. The rest of us is trained to sit still. In addition, for some of us, religious tradition has fostered soul-body separation and directed us to subdue bodily explorations and pleasures. If we participate in athletics, often a no-pain-no-gain mentality pushes us to "train" the body rather than appreciate and learn from it. With the preponderance of screen watching, physical "fitness" is now often reduced to channel switching and occasional trips to the kitchen for the three C's of body abuse: cola, chips, and chocolate.

Even within these limitations, the body continues to store up experiences. Fumes from a father's beer belch as he curses the referee's call are remembered by the son perched alongside his dad, especially if oft-repeated, and so is the child's resulting agitation or pleasure. That smell forever stirs up the same set of sensations and sentiments, even when that child has become an old man.

For me, writing the word "valley" brings a slight flush to my cheeks and a tightness to my forehead. Embodied in me still is the memory of my fifth-grade classmates' cheers and mocking laughter when I failed to win the annual spelling championship. I was getting my comeuppance for my snobby attitude when I outlasted the competition in previous years. *How could I, living in the town of Valley City, have been so stupid!?*

So powerful is the embodiment of our history that it is common for children to sound and walk a lot like their parents, and even to acquire the same illnesses—the result of more than genetic legacy. Nonfamilial regional similarities confirm that the body absorbs and expresses what's familiar. Note the preponderance of fast-talking, arm-flailing New Yorkers versus staid Midwestern slow talkers.

Yet, what is so familiar is oddly strange to us as well. We don't notice the shape we're in until our bodies plead in pain. Constrained conditioning has made us into somatic illiterates. After living in our bodies for all these years, we hardly know them. We've learned to regard them as servants rather than as intimates. We expect them to do our mind's bidding and to hold up well regardless of how we treat them. It's rare that we stop to make their acquaintance and find out what they know or desire.

Around age fifty, I noticed spots in front of my eyes as I was reading. From an ophthamologist I learned that they're called "floaters." Sure that this problem could be repaired, I asked what could be done. Nothing, I was told. "It's a temporary condition, but it's one that comes with aging," he said. No one had ever used the word "aging" about me before. I couldn't hear anything else the doctor said. Around this same time, hot flashes began, and memory lapses became apparent. "The change," it's called, but it wasn't the only change I was experiencing. Long-standing neck and shoulder tightness, years of repetitive keyboarding, thousands of awkward tennis swings, and a history of posture neglect, among other bad habits, were leaving pain, stiffness, and limited mobility. Ice packs, elbow wraps, and soothing balms began taking up space in my household cabinets, and I became a frequent client of chiropractors, physical therapists, and massage therapists. The body I had taken for granted, the body I had given little attention, except for a halfhearted exercise routine, now demanded a great deal of care.

My response was mostly in the "repair and rescue" mode: Let's get this thing working again as fast as possible—and back in service!

I had a similar response to the panic attacks I was experiencing and to the stomach tension, ankle swelling, and myriad other signals that seemed like perturbing shrieks of an unruly child. Okay, I'll change diet and lifestyle, listen to relaxation tapes, practice deep breathing—whatever it takes to stave off this surge of physical rebellion. Added to my to-do list was body mending.

In a painting class in my early twenties, the teacher gave us an assignment to go outside and lie on our bellies in the grass for ten minutes and peer with curious eyes at what lay before us. Never before had I been exposed to the intricate life of the soil. Each tiny lump of dirt had its own shape, color, and light patterns. Sculpting it from below were roots pushing up infant shoots. Slow-moving and darting insects—black, gray, brown, red, green—climbed and crawled, adding to the sculpture with their minute lifting, flicking, and shoving. Each grass blade displayed its particular size, curve, hue, and wave with the wind. When I rose from the ground, I knew that piece of land and its story like a lover knows the face of the beloved. I had attended to its astonishing beauty and mysteries as an intimate witness. I could paint it now, but more important, I was no longer apart from it. It wasn't just the ground upon which I walked; I had entered its story and its story had entered mine.

In a similar vein, I have gotten to know my body through the Feldenkrais Method, a set of movement-learning practices developed by Israeli physicist and martial arts master Moshe Feldenkrais. Using tiny, easygoing movements, a Feldenkrais lesson (done with the help of a practitioner, book, or recorded guidance) invites microscopic observation of how a hand goes through the process of opening and closing or of how much farther one shoulder or hip rotates than the other. Through this close-up study, I am able to explore intricately how I move and hold my body and what those patterns tell me about my (often unconscious) ways of relating and taking action.

In doing Feldenkrais lessons, I become again like the art student "watching" in awe, but with more engagement, using my inside senses of movement, balance, and spatial awareness. In some of the lessons, I rediscover the pleasure of rolling and stretching and turning in ways forgotten since infancy. In some cases, I learn what somehow I missed as a baby. And I gain heightened awareness of my pervasive tendencies, conditioned after decades of practice. In one lesson that I especially enjoy, my body reports to me how I move quickly from one activity to another in my life, and I am gently reintroduced to the pleasure of allowing time for *completion*. Whenever I finish a Feldenkrais lesson, I feel intimately at home inside my skin.

It doesn't take elaborate instructions, however, to make such intimate acquaintance. In a course I teach on body awareness, one week's homework assignment is to find a new way to play. One woman in the class, who had a delightfully bold and quirky personality, chose as her new activity to relearn what she had done easily as an infant—getting her big toe all the way to her mouth!

Why not? Is there any reason to stay "out of touch"? Or maybe the better question might be: Is there something to be gained from getting in touch—literally—with our bodies, enjoying them as a playground, exploring their history and their mysteries? I think there is.

My experience with Cherie blowing the lid off my kidnapping experience was life-changing. I learned at a cellular level that the body "knows" things that I often try to hide from or simply don't notice. With practice, I am learning that the more I listen to it, the more my aliveness grows. Before meeting Cherie, I had considered that encounter with my kidnapper as a sacred one. I still do, because of the spiritual strength I found in its midst and because of the wonder of this young man's loving response from his jail cell. But, so deeply was I enamored with the spiritual that I unwittingly sustained the soul-body duality of my religious upbringing, ignoring and thus suppressing my visceral responses. After the kidnapping experience, I never adequately acknowledged the intense fear and anger trapped inside of me—the natural biological response of terror and outrage built in for my own self-protection under serious threat. I had "spiritualized" that away. My body, though, hadn't forgotten. Long after Larry released me from captivity, my body had kept my fear and fury in holding cells until five years later when I could feel safe enough to discharge them.

In Cherie's presence, where I had come ready to free up unexplained body tensions and where I felt total acceptance, I found support for embracing and then freeing the remnants of the kidnapping that still held me captive. I was able to express feelings that weren't "nice," parting from the stringent mores of my German Catholic upbringing. I didn't feel the need to be strong or "good" with Cherie, or even loving—except toward myself. I was able to enter a new, more integrated domain, recognizing through an embodied experience that I could claim my fear and anger without destroying or condemning myself and without losing my ability to understand and forgive my kidnapper. It's a lesson I am still refining.

This was not my first body lesson nor the first time I grasped the need to honor the full array of my emotions. But its intensity provoked a lasting and insatiable curiosity about the wonders our bodies contain. It also provoked a sadness about how much we lose touch with our bodies as we move from babyhood to adulthood. In my early sixties, I'm only now getting glimpses of what's been lost to me over my lifetime, including the relief of shedding tears when good friends died, because I had deeply absorbed a shaming childhood message that only "big babies" cry.

I am not alone in what I've lost. Many massage therapists and other bodyworkers can tell of clients' long-held tears being released or memories of forgotten abuse surfacing when their bodies' suppressed emotions were awakened through touch. Joys, too, are suppressed for some people who were told as children "Don't be silly" or "Grow up!" Many children of alcoholics or ill parents had to assume adult responsibilities at a young age in order to take care of their parents. They had so little opportunity to enjoy the pleasures of childhood that they literally have to be taught how to play in adulthood.

Even beyond the losses that many people experience as the result of such traumas, the bigger loss for all of us is the lasting imprint from our cultural history of dismissal and distancing from our bodies. We don't feel at home in our bodies much; often, we're at war with them. In addition, we are deluged with commercial messages that tell us our bodies aren't satisfactory and need to be tucked, indulged, thinned, or medicated. As the average age of the population mounts, the body is becoming even more of an enemy. Wrinkles and joint pains frighten baby boomers. A massive fight-or-flight response to body changes prevails. The aging body is feared and shunned. Witness the abundance of anti-aging creams created to help erase the face of aging, and the glee expressed when an older person is praised for youthful appearance. What might the aging body teach us if, instead of trying to negate it or bring it under control, we decided to explore its riches?

Our bodies are rich resources at any age. But by the second half of our lives, we have more experience to draw on. Millions of moments of living are packed into our somatic storehouses—a wealth of potential enjoyment, wisdom, learning, and creativity. Rather than Botoxing or fortifying our bodies in an effort to look and feel younger, it might be more satisfying to give them fresh and mindful attention in order to notice what they have to offer, so we can make ourselves at home in them. They are already talking to us anyway through our aches and pains, our edginess and fatigue, our urges and surges. One way or another, our bodies' stories will be told, as my encounter with Cherie surely testifies. If we listen carefully, our bodies may take us beyond the feared notions of decline, decrepitude, and death.

Every session of a six-week course I teach starts with the participants standing in a circle, playing catch with a colorful ball. Lively music helps to set the pace and spirit of the activity. The course, called Writing Your Own Permission Slip, is designed to draw on the wisdom and aliveness of our bodies to prompt transformative personal writing. In each session, we move and play and attend to our bodies in a variety of ways. The physical activity stimulates awareness, memory, and creativity. In the first session, for example, we say our names as we toss the ball, first in our normal voices, and then in a variety of playful ways, such as with the tone of voice used by our parents when they called us in from playing outside. Once this physical romp opens our unconscious storehouse of embodied memories, writing exercises help us reinvent our self-definitions.

Most people who take this course are in their fifties or older. Ray, age seventy, a thin, stiff-bodied, retired engineer with a severe hearing loss, signed up seeking relief from his depression. He was feeling overwhelmed and defeated in the face of his wife's Alzheimer's. Sara, a short, talkative, mid-fifties woman with an angelic face, was easily moved to tears and laughter.

She had spent a year in intense grieving after nursing her husband through the dying process and wanted to find a way to move on. Lola, eighty-eight, was a bright-faced, glamorously dressed elf. She came to the class "to find my purpose," she said, and was eager to do more creative writing. Paul was seventy. A tall man, he was slow to speak and flat-voiced, but eloquent. A composer of choral music, he wanted to recapture flagging zest and creativity.

Through physical play, coupled with imagination and writing exercises, these course participants unveiled memories and desires embedded in their cells. Ray reconnected with the joy of playing a musical instrument remembered from his childhood; he decided to take guitar lessons. Sara soon found a way to turn her attention beyond grief to begin a new life. She rediscovered lessons of courage and resilience from a class exercise in which she was asked to pay attention to the wisdom of an old scar on her body. Lola, when assigned a leading role as angel-guide in a dramatization, exercised her creative wit and reignited her purpose of joyously giving to others. Lola also reactivated lost physical abilities, including being able to catch a ball. Paul found delight in replaying a boyhood game (catch) and in dramatizing a jungle scene in which he played a friendly lion on all fours, roar and all. Soon afterward, with his imagination rekindled, he invited the other course participants to a premiere performance of his newest choral piece.

In this course, the personal myths by which older participants such as these are living—common myths about aging in America today—get revised as they tune in to their bodies in new ways. Their body wisdom, combined with their imagination, springs them free from wasteland images of aging.

What would happen if all of us viewed our aging, not primarily as a time of deterioration and detriment, but of revelation? Our experience of aging might become not one of diminishment but of discovery. Let's face it: most of us are going to live longer than our parents did, a lot longer. Since we've never been old before, perhaps we could enter our older years with the same curiosity and sense of wonder as two-year-olds who have never experienced childhood before. Perhaps there is not so much to fear as there is to learn. Whether we attend body-oriented workshops and classes, perform simple acts of mindful attention, or choose other ways of somatic exploration, our bodies are treasure chests of our past and windows into our present. When we value our bodies as ongoing personal resources for self-discovery and creativity, they can become our guides throughout our lives. What delight may await us if we listen to them pour out their stories—*our* stories.

Chapter Three

Turning 50

*B*y the time I was approaching fifty, I had only begun to awaken to the stories my body had to tell. In some ways, my body was coaxing me to listen, even demanding to be heard. An assortment of aches, a reinvigorated sexuality as I began dating following my divorce, and a burgeoning restlessness all beckoned me.

About that time, it also dawned on me that I might live to be a hundred. This was both shocking and exciting. Until then, I realized, life had mostly happened *to* me; I'd lived primarily in a reaction mode. My mother's cautionary "Be careful" and "What will people think?" had been my guarded guidance, along with my religion's "Be ye perfect." While I had chosen whom to marry and what careers to follow, generally my goal had been to figure out how to get along, win approval, and get things right. My body had been sculpted to fit all these constraints—forced smile, tense shoulders, tucked-in chest, stiff back, tightly held hips.

With the prospect of fifty-plus years before me, I wondered about the power and possibility of living fully from choice rather than reaction, of living from the inside out. I decided I wanted to go about creating the second half of my life with intention and declaration. Instead of being acceptable or right, I wanted to be playful, curious, and bold. This was more than a decision of the mind. A feverish fermenting was taking place, a thrust of energy pushing up through my core. My whole being was yearning to *move*, to *generate*.

When I planned my fiftieth birthday party, more than anything else I wanted to include African dancing. In my limited exposure to this ancient way of moving, I had been drawn by its fluid yet declarative pulsing that seemed earthbound, yet boundless. I also wanted the party held at a place where I could play out under the stars. I wanted infinite room to move. Only people I thought were willing to be outrageous were invited. Maggie Kuhn, founder of the Gray Panther Party, had become my role model with her commitment to doing something outrageous every day. With the promise of fifty years of outrageous living ahead of me, I wanted to get off to a good start. My body was craving to take the lead.

When I imagined which friends and acquaintances might freely let loose with African rhythms, the invitation list was disappointingly small. Had I really accumulated such a cautious, restrained group of friends? Only a couple of those who attended actually set down their wine glasses and plates of nibblies and joined me in letting the music shake and sway the pelvis. None of us were trained dancers, and only a few had even witnessed African dance, but I had hoped for an evening of playfully breaking free from restraints. I trusted the music to teach my body how to move. My first lesson in outrageous living was that hope wasn't sufficient. Neither was waiting for someone else to create the dance.

With high-volume, pounding drumbeats of Suru Ekeh's "Witch Doctor" pouring out of the speakers, I stepped into the center of the room. Not like the sixteen-year-old I once was with straggly ponytail, bulky glasses, and rounded shoulders, standing shyly along the edge of the dance floor, forcing a smile and longing for even a glance from a boy. Not like the once-wife I had been for more than two decades, who, though assured of a dance partner, was still not looked at. No, I was creating rather than waiting. My hips, which had practiced holding and hoping for too long, began to roll forward, back, forward, back. Shoulders folded toward the chest as the lower back rounded and then thrust upward with royal claim, filling out my torso's undulation. Knees and toes alternated inward and out as my feet leapt lightly with the rhythm of the drums. The ebb and flow of living waters, the sparking of passionate fires, the earth's pulsing heartbeat, and the free flowing of breath all claimed me. I was being moved and consumed by fresh but ancient forces, swirling me inward and outward and homeward amidst smoke from damp kindling. Surrendering to the elements and to the sensual, my whole body softened.

A friend who shared my birth date stepped forward, willing to enter with me into the rhythmic mysteries and mercies of living water, earth, wind, and fire. Eye-to-eye we danced, losing ourselves in a timeless gaze, letting our bodies roll and sway and brush against each other in movements that had now gone beyond ethnic origins to universal waves and pulsations. My palm against his, we were sweeping upward, then twirling around back to back, and turning again to let our legs and arms intersect, and continuing in a flow of gyrations that whispered of male and female honoring rather than seduction. This was a night of creation, a birthing ceremony for the next fifty years.

In adulthood, it's all too rare that we let our bodies lead us into primal and playful creations without restraint. That's especially true as we get older. In early adulthood, it's acceptable to romp around on the floor with our kids and to dance to a raucous beat on Saturday night. But many adult physical activities are dictated by preset forms—the rules of a sport, a set of exercises for our health, or even the routine moves to complete household or workplace tasks. As we advance in age, even parties often turn into stand-up cocktail affairs, potluck eating fests, or gatherings around a screen for shared viewing. How few are the opportunities for freewheeling movement, for letting the body be adventurously expressive. When so much of our day-to-day tension, and even pain, results from repetitive, constricted motions, couldn't more of our leisure activities be directed to giving us free rein? Couldn't social proprieties be abandoned now and then, without the need to rely on a few drinks to "loosen us up"? Maybe that's why there's been an upswing of interest in adventure travel. People may crave kayaking on the Amazon or scrambling up Andean passes in part simply so their bodies can indulge in moves that their everyday lives don't allow.

Sometimes a distinctive milestone, like a decade birthday or an illness or a moment of great soulfulness, compels us to make a dramatic expression in physical form. Sherri, a Jewish preschool teacher and friend of mine, nervously took her first international trip at age forty-nine, traveling with a friend to Israel, where she had longed to go for years. It was a pilgrimage of sorts, to find her way back to where she had come from. On a mountaintop at Qumran, overlooking a vast spread of desert, she felt a strange and pressing desire—to remove her blouse and bra and raise her arms to the sky. "It was so uncommon for me to even think of doing something like that," she told me with a sheepish grin, but then her smile quickly widened and she became gleeful as she went on, "I just had to do it. I don't know why. It was something about being there, feeling so at one with nature. There was nothing sexual about it, I just wanted to feel the freedom, and I did. It was wonderful." This was a holy moment for her—not the kind she had expected on this trip. It was a return to the homeland of her body. To help her remember, she asked her friend to snap a photo of her from the back, with her armed stretched skyward. But even if she lost track of the photo, I can imagine that her body feels different to her now, more her own. I have secretly wished for a long time that I could spend a time in a beautiful place outdoors bare-breasted. The time may come for me as it did for Sherri, when I just have to do it.

Our bodies are remarkably inventive at revealing what's stirring inside us and what's in need of healing. Undeniable physical urges spurred me to attempt African dancing so I could slither out of my wallflower skin, long overdue its shedding. An irresistible impulse nudged Sherri to discard her customary coverings. There comes a moment of maturity, confidence, inspiration, or safety, where the holding on or holding back just seems useless, even silly. The body's memories or urges emerge unbidden, erupting simply because it's time.

The grassy area beside the farmhouse of my childhood slopes for a dozen yards or so down toward the driveway, and I rolled down it any number of times in my early years. I'd position myself sideways, give my shoulders and hips a starter thrust, and then gravity would take charge, flipping and flopping my body over and over, flinging me at dizzying speed. Again and again on a summer's day, I would scramble to the top of the incline and tumble my way down to the bottom with abandon, spinning and squealing out of control. Even at age sixteen there were days of summer boredom when the thrill of the hill still seduced me. But one day a cramping pain stabbed me halfway through a roll. I stopped awkwardly and curled up, puzzled, changed. Soon after, what I saw for the first time was blood between my legs.

It was time to enter womanhood now, to hold myself erect, to mount high heels, to tuck in my tummy, to hide my bloodiness, to keep my behavior under control. Boys turning into men could still toss balls and tumble around on the ground; girls turning women were to watch and cheer. I never rolled down that hill again.

I didn't quit being a "tomboy" altogether, and I regained many lost body freedoms over the years as I joined other women in claiming our right to move as we choose. But I'd never gone down a hill again, the way I did as a child. And I wanted to.

From the time I turned fifty and my bleeding stopped, I kept my eye open for a rolling hill like that one—a good-sized hill slanted just right and padded with thick grass. I've seen some and felt the longing to roll there, but I always passed on by. A foolish thing, I thought. People would see me. I'm not dressed for it. Another time.

I remembered a perfect hill one day, one I'd often passed. I smiled and felt a whoosh of adrenaline as I imagined reliving the long-ago thrill of free rolling, but I couldn't quite imagine going to this hill at my age and actually doing what I dreamed. Besides, the hill was near a walking trail and lots of dogs are let loose to romp there. Still, I wanted to roll once more. Maybe there's another hill like this, I started to imagine, one secluded enough for a private tumble, but I soon dismissed the thought. *Such silliness*, I heard my mother's voice echo through me.

One evening I went off on a bike ride with the idea of wanting to find a fresh way to play. (I had given that assignment to a class I was teaching, and I always do the assignments myself.) I veered off my usual route onto a short side trail that I knew dead-ended in a small woody area. As I rode along, I glanced to one side and saw a very narrow and steep hill, one that appeared to have been deliberately built from piled-up loads of dirt as if intended for dirt bike runs or winter sledding. I remembered seeing it the last time I'd been this way, but it newly caught my eye. Its fairly even surface, covered in grass, beckoned now as an ideal spot for rolling.

But I hadn't planned to roll, not tonight. I'd look foolish if anyone saw me. Again, *such silliness.* Still, this was an out-of-the-way place with little chance of anyone spotting me. Unable to convince myself, I passed on by, biking on to a little-used ballpark around the back side of the hill—an even more remote location. Maybe I could do my rolling on this side of the hill, I thought for a moment, but I quickly rationalized that it was too secluded if I got hurt while rolling.

I made a U-turn to head back, thinking, well, maybe yes, I would actually go for it. Yes, I'd roll down the front side of the hill before heading home. This would be my "new" way to play—at least a way I'd never played as a grown-up. Heading back around the hill, ready for my adventure, I was wearing a silly grin and feeling nervous.

Darn! Three kids were circling around on bikes near the bottom of the hill. *Well, what if I invited them to roll with me?* For a moment, I actually entertained that idea, but soon dismissed it as only a storybook notion, then watched as they quickly biked out of sight.

Now's my chance. Here's the hill I've wanted. Why wait?

I parked my bike and mounted the hill quickly. After taking one more look around to make sure no one was in sight, I lay on my side and started to roll—cautiously. After a few turns, I stopped. *Can I really do this? Yes. I must. Go!* Another half dozen spins and I could tell I was headed not down the hill but at an angle, rolling off to one side. Stopping again, I repositioned myself, pushed off, and rolled unhindered, body flipping and flopping fast, head spinning, stomach spinning, eyes sighting sky, grass, sky, grass, sky. *Omigod, what if there are sharp rocks or big bumps?* I tried to look up to check but instantly felt the added strain on my neck from rolling in this cockeyed position. I succumbed at last to the spinning, safe or not, and I rolled on and on and on all the way to the bottom—out of control.

No mother voice was stopping me now. There were no social mores to follow, no one to please or impress. It wasn't dignified. It wasn't pretty. But it was *me*—giving myself over to my own momentum, helped along by the forces of mother earth, giving in to freedom. I felt like Sam Keen, the trapeze novice at age sixty-one, who, when he couldn't seem to bring himself through a successful leap to the next swing one day, decided instead that it was a good day to practice falling. The only measure of success was the willingness to let go and enjoy the descent.

Sprawled at the bottom of the hill, I was relieved to find I was still breathing—and felt no big pain. The ground beneath me felt firm and stable. The sky was still swirling past me rapidly, so I closed my eyes. I felt a little nauseous and was suddenly achy in many places. Two or three minutes passed before I made my way to standing. On unsteady feet, I wobbled toward my bike.

After checking to see if each body part still worked as usual, I mounted the bike in slow motion. As I pressed on the pedal, a slight pain pinged momentarily through my right foot. My left knee felt slightly out of joint, so I shook it a little. *There!* It was all right.

Assured that I was safe and barely damaged, I smiled to myself and took a deep breath. I briefly looked back at the hill I had just conquered, not by arduous climbing to achieve some feat of endurance, but by letting myself surrender. I wished for a moment that someone had been there to watch, to say, "Good for you" or to laugh with me at my cautions and clumsiness. Then I wondered if anyone would think I was silly or crazy if I told them what I'd done. But I quickly dismissed these outdated concerns. *What does it matter?* I had simply done what I had longed to do for a very long time. I had rolled down a big hill, just like when I was a kid. *Such silliness,* indeed! Such fun!

The Body as Metaphor and Mirror

*L*ike good literature, the body sometimes speaks through metaphor. Somatic clues abound that reveal the nature of internal disturbances of mind and soul. Neck muscles tense. A rash breaks out. Feet swell. Such physical disturbances could merely be the result of something we ate or a pollutant in the environment or the side effect of a drug, and if so, we can make necessary adjustments to feel better again. But maybe the body's distress signal is a long-suffering call of desperation expressed as metaphor. Who or what has become a "pain in the neck"? What in us wants to break out—or what poison are we're trying to expel? What is feeling so large and weighted within us that our feet can't move forward?

A delightful and wise friend of mine knew I'd been struggling mightily with a simple task—getting an appointment set with a colleague in order to meet a work deadline. In the midst of this struggle, I had a tooth pulled because of a persistent infection. My friend suggested to me that maybe now, with the tooth gone, "You will no longer have to feel like you're pulling teeth." We both laughed at the metaphor; it was surely apt. Had I noted it earlier, perhaps the humor in it might have served as an antibiotic for my persistent tendency to turn my work into *hard* work.

James Hillman, in *The Force of Character and the Lasting Life*, reflects on the archetypal meaning of symptoms and problems, especially those that the aging body reveals. He suggests radical metaphorical understandings of such changes as the slowing and drying and sagging of the body. "Are we merely turning into juiceless mummies with parchment skin?" he asks. No, he says, the dry body is reflective of the "dry soul," transformed by the alchemy of age through "evaporation [that] lets off the steam [and] boils away the moisture that has kept you stuck." It is freed of the "messy, sticky situations" of heavy emotional involvement that saturate much of our lives. "Too much liquid and the soul substance tends to putrefy. You feel yourself swamped, flooded; can't get out of this mood; stagnating." Hillman speaks of the emotion being "extracted" in this alchemical process until it becomes merely an "interesting curiosity." He says, "The reduction of the past to dry facts yields the salt wisdom that the old are supposedly able to dispense." Using another metaphorical mélange, he suggests that aged ones "are the light keepers, the enlighteners whose wisdom can see into the dark. Their characters must carry a fire. Therefore they must be dry."

Metaphors can be clarifying windows into the body's presentation of itself. Hannah's intestinal disturbances made sense when Cherie McCoy helped her pay close attention to what she couldn't "stomach." Stooped shoulders might suggest someone who wears the world as a heavy burden. One older woman in my Writing Your Own Permission Slip course kept commenting before the class began that she was "scared stiff." Hers was a stick-stiff torso, already speaking of her internal constrictions before she voiced them. Our bodies are our outerwear, shaped by our experience and our perspectives—and also shapers of them. The stiff woman, after several rounds of tossing, kicking, and catching balls during the class, reinvigorated the gleeful playfulness of her childhood. When it came time for her to write, she served up images of carefree swinging and romping through backyards. Her body's experience awakened a new metaphor.

Sometimes the metaphors need to be coaxed out. This may take time. If I feel discomfort in my body, I usually want to relieve the discomfort—fast! If I've got a swollen knee or digestive difficulties, forget looking for significance, I've got things to do, let's just get this problem fixed. In the same way, when I am reading books or magazines, I've conditioned myself to skip over the stories or pictures and get to the author's main point. I want information and solutions. Who's got time for meandering tales? Just tell me what I need to know or do. Our high-speed world has encoded in me a drive for efficiency that too often starves me of the nourishment and pleasures of images and stories. I miss the wisdom for the facts.

As I've gotten older, however, I've become more willing to linger, and stories interest me more. Sometimes the story is all I need to know; it's often a metaphor with the message built in. When I allow myself to sink into a worthy story, it enfolds me, cocoons me, nurturing a new tale within me that is ready to take wing.

That same lingering listening serves me well when I become aware of a body ailment, a posture I'm holding, or a physical reaction to something that happens. If I have soreness in my wrists, a tight jaw, or a rapid heartbeat when threatened, what analogy will reveal itself, what metaphor emerge, if I become as curious as a child? The metaphor that enlightens me may be in the body's condition itself, or something around me may offer an image reflecting and thus clarifying what I'm experiencing in my body.

In my Permission Slip class, I ask students to write one hundred different responses to the sentence fragment "Sometimes my life is like . . ." Typically, students find the first dozen or two comparisons easy to come up with; they are often clichéd: "Sometimes my life is like . . . a roller coaster . . . a speedboat . . . a race against time." Once these worn images are exhausted and another seventy or more must be created, the students dig deeper inside themselves and the real discovery begins: "Sometimes my life is like . . . a TV with too many channels . . . a cradle waiting to rock me . . . a Buick with the horsepower of a little red wagon." A hundred similes reveal a gallery of images ripe for prompting self-awareness, experimentation, and make-believe.

When I do the exercise myself, I try to be censor-free, writing rapidly whatever comes to mind. Some images on my list are more or less meaningless, but then there are those that I *feel;* something in my body says *Yes!* When I wrote, "Sometimes my life is like standing behind a lectern too tall for me," I immediately felt *small, shrunken.* I could literally sense my body dropping its weight and curling over slightly. I felt like I was six, having just strained on tiptoes to be seen and then collapsed in embarrassment after realizing I wasn't grown up enough to be speaking at big lecterns before audiences. Then more sensations emerged—the expressionless face, tightened tummy, rapid heartbeat, and motionless torso I exhibit sometimes even now when speaking onstage. I became aware that I wasn't feeling very "grown up" in those moments (or overall in my professional life) at that particular time in my life. I had tried to cover that up, but this simile unveiled how my body was holding these hidden fears of incompetence and looking foolish. As I took time to observe and appreciate the body sensations and emotions coaxed out by this simile, I had compassion for that shrunken, embarrassed one still needing assurance, and I begin to help her feel safe again. Knowing that my body carries an entire archive of experiences, I looked for other similes on my list that might be equally revealing and call forth more confident somatic responses: "Sometimes my life is like a playground . . . a dancing studio . . . a science lab with experiments going on all over the place . . . a game of Let's Play Queen."

Maybe next time I do the exercise, I will start with "Sometimes

my body is like . . ." or "my sore elbow is like . . ." or "my ar-
thritic hand is like . . ." Who knows what my body might tell
me if I gave it the chance to imagine itself in a hundred different
ways?

The mind expresses itself through the body, and the body becomes the messenger to those around as well as to the person
within. Intense or long-buried emotional or mental distress, in
particular, often shows up in physical forms that are metaphori-
cally loaded. What's "eating" someone, for example, may at first
gnaw away at her insides, creating a roiling stomach or some
other internal disturbance. But if the disturbance becomes too
tumultuous or venomous to tolerate, the person might expel it
in a combined physical and metaphorical form through spitting
or vomiting, or perhaps through venomous behavior. The metaphor may also be projected onto an external object or person.

Martín Prechtel, a shaman of Guatemalan heritage, told me
a story of an experience he had with a man who attended one
of his personal enrichment weekends. The man began to run
around, yelling and acting wildly, declaring he had poisoned the
bagels that the participants were eating. The other people were
understandably disturbed. But Prechtel began to talk with the
man and soon learned that the "poison" was, in fact, his "contempt" for certain things that were deeply troubling to him. The
risk-encouraging, yet supportive nature of the weekend had evidently created enough safety for this man to unleash his back-
log of bottled-up fury and disgust, albeit in an unfriendly form.
Once his body didn't have to hold it in anymore, it came out
as a kind of foaming at the mouth. Just as I couldn't control my
fierce trembling in my experience with Cherie, this ranting man
apparently had little or no control over his bizarre behavior.
Yet, even in this emboldened state, he externalized part of his
feelings in the "poisoned" bagels. In my case, the sound of the

crashing chair had been an unbidden projection of my pain, instigating my "out of control" behavior; in his case, the external point of projection was a specific food item he chose. *Perhaps* he chose it, that is. Or, perhaps it, too, had a relevant and compelling association in his memory bank—maybe some "poisonous" or "contemptible" eating experience from his past.

Prechtel continued to eat his "poisoned" bagel, telling the man, "I want to see what your contempt tastes like." Prechtel was unafraid of the man's craziness and wanted to "taste" it, to understand it. He modeled for the man the possibility of tasting the contempt for himself—with appreciation and a calm curiosity—rather than continuing to turn it into a destructive force, internally or externally. With further support during the weekend, the man was able to calm his tantrum-like behavior and give voice to his long-buried pain in less harmful ways, so he could learn from it and become free of it.

In a similar case, Evelyn, a hospital nurse, told me about her success in dealing with a particularly difficult patient—a Vietnam veteran suffering from post-traumatic stress disorder. Other nurses were highly frustrated by his frequent outbursts of terror when the remnants of wartime trauma, so deeply embedded in his somatic structures, convinced him that he was again under enemy attack. The nurses couldn't get close enough to administer his medication, let alone do routine blood pressure checks. Evelyn won his cooperation by joining in his drama with full vigor, getting down under the bed alongside him and yelling, "Keep your head down. Don't move or they'll hear us." Staying in character, she guided him safely out of his state of siege. Because she became his ally, he allowed her to carry out necessary medical procedures.

Like Prechtel, Evelyn was willing to meet and taste the experience of the person in pain—to physically enter inside the person's metaphor, not for the purpose of sharing in the suffering, but to acknowledge its presence and its power. This willingness to "get physical" resulted in gaining the person's trust. It was a way to help the healing begin.

Wise healers like Prechtel and Evelyn are attentive to metaphorical clues, whether their physical form is only felt somatically or (as in the above cases) it's also expressed behaviorally. They follow these clues until they find a way to demonstrate that they are looking through the eyes or tasting the pain of the afflicted. By visiting or mirroring the wounded person's worldview in a physical manner (since it's expressed physically), they can then more easily help the person to adjust the distortions and take in a more balanced version of reality.

These healers are instructive in their methods. Like them, we can all find our own way to a wider and saner reality if we listen attentively to what our bodies reveal and give the message due acknowledgment. For example, I've become aware that I often walk around with my head thrust forward slightly ahead of the rest of my body. When I notice I'm doing it, I can usually pick up on how rushed I'm feeling—to "get things done." Other body tensions also become apparent. This simple act of awareness—the stopping of the action to pay curious attention—is often enough to dissolve the distress.

Sometimes it's a clue in the environment that leads to understanding a physical disturbance, especially if it has an emotional underpinning. What is happening around me points to, or amplifies, what is going on inwardly—and becomes the mirror inviting awareness and healing. The mirror might reflect either my problems or my desires. A purring kitten can be a mirror reflecting my desire for relaxation—and quickly prompt a bodily response of calm. Seeing a speeding car get into a crash might alert me to my own overly high-speed pace that's got me "crashing" into people in my life instead of cruising alongside them.

I struggled with the "hard work" project in part because I was in the midst of a short period of depression—close to despair. I couldn't clearly identify the source of this desolate state of mind, but as the depression mounted, I felt less and less confident and more and more incapable of getting things done. The depression played out physically as very low energy, a somber facial expression, a flat voice, and a feeling of heaviness. Despite taking St. John's wort, exercising, watching funny movies, and other attempts at endorphin stimulation, everything felt like an effort.

At the height of my anguish, I was preparing one night for a class session of a graduate writing course I was teaching. As I looked over the three manuscripts students had submitted for critiquing, I was jarred by their uncanny similarity in themes: the first was on depression, the second on suicide, the third on death.

I stared for several minutes at this hall of mirrors, my eyes and jaws widening as I pondered its meaning. Had my own state of mind and body become a magnet for this grim collection, I wondered—like attracting like? Just the thought of this possibility landed forty pounds of coal on my chest. I sank back into my rocking chair. My breathing stopped. But only for a moment. In mind-body syncopation, I reacted mightily to this pressed-down sensation. I remember thinking, *If collecting such dour tales bodes what's in store in my depressed state, I'd better snap out of it!* I also thought, *If I am powerful enough to draw to myself such deadly reinforcing reflections, then I'm also powerful enough to attract ones that are more life-giving. But, to do that, I'd have to shift out of my depressed state.* Of course, I couldn't know in any logically objective way if this triple magnifier of manuscripts was more than a coincidence, but my gut response to it was immediate. Even the prospect of having some kind of power over my environment jolted through me like an energy charge, igniting neuronal sparks throughout my torso, sitting me up straighter, loosening my taut neck muscles. As if the coal had landed on a keg of dynamite, the lighted fuse inside of me prompted its quick and dramatic detonation. This full-bodied moment of recognition was so startling that my hand felt propelled to reach for the phone so I could share the news. I burst into laughter as I told a friend how "powerful" I was. That moment was the beginning of the turnaround in my ability to get the appointment set with my work colleague and meet the deadline. And the depression lifted soon after.

I doubt that the similarity of themes in those manuscripts had any intrinsic significance. But I—mind and body—made meaning from it. The amplification of my depression as I saw it mirrored in triplicate showed me where I was headed and scared me into changing course. This was partly a mental re-action, but my body's response was equally potent: it wasn't willing to bear the weight of sinking any lower into its already oppressive state of misery. A basic biological survival instinct kicked in. The neuronal ignition and adrenaline rush I was feel-ing were allowing me to fight for my life. Looking in the mirror had saved me.

My body often picks up on clues like these in my environ-ment, even before my mind does. It is drawn to situations or things that, through mirroring, create an impetus toward re-solving its distress or satisfying its wants. Or, sometimes the mirror just calls forth stories wanting to be remembered—and revised or retold.

§ Chapter Five

No Brakes

*T*hat was my immediate conclusion: no brakes. My car was moving forward and I couldn't stop it. There was a minivan stopped in front of me at the intersection. My foot reached for the brake pedal as always. Automatic. Touch the brake pedal, the car slows. Push harder on the brake pedal, the car stops. I had done it thousands of time, and every time before it had worked. I had come to depend on my brakes. They were as certain as gravity. Whenever I raise a foot to take a step forward, gravity tugs it back downward. I can count on it. So, I stepped on the brake. When the automatic response wasn't there, I quickly tried again. No response. The car continued to move ahead. In that moment, my attention became riveted on stopping the car. I barely noticed the deep breaths of my passengers. I pushed again, hard, with all the strength in my foot, my leg, my middle. No response. I gave both feet to the effort. This time I pushed with all my strength. Every muscle in my body strained, right up through my forehead. My entire body was elongated, my bottom raised off the seat, my shoulders jammed against the seat back. I generated a surge of strength that felt powerful enough to stop a train. I was giving it all I had. It wasn't enough. The car continued easing forward, unaffected by my posture, my determination, or my trust.

The van grew in height and girth as we neared it. We would be merging with it. There was nowhere to turn away, and no time. I tried to look away, but my body was *so sure* it could make the car stop. It *had* to make the car stop. It had always worked before. *If I pushed hard enough, the car would stop.* Yet I already knew it wouldn't. I already knew that what I had relied on all of my life with total trust was not reliable now. I had done all the right things, and they hadn't worked. No amount of continuing to do those "right things" was going to make a difference. I was powerless. We were going to crash no matter what I did. *The car was out of my control.*

I had one final hope. The car wasn't going very fast—maybe fifteen to twenty miles per hour. Maybe it would stop on its own, simply because I wasn't applying the gas. Or maybe the van would move away just in time. Something had to work here. This just couldn't be happening.

Nothing helped. Not all my efforts nor all my certainty nor all my hope. My car's bumper connected with the van's. It was over. For a few moments, my body remained frozen in its strained, outstretched position, feet still firmly planted on the brake pedal. Then, I put the car in park and stepped out of the door.

It quickly became apparent that the collision had been quite minor, barely felt by me and my passengers. The only obvious damage was to my license plate and its holder. It also became quickly apparent that the source of the problem was not my brakes, but a small patch of clear ice so unexpected on a sunny April afternoon despite some last-blast-of-winter blustery snow earlier in the day. It was just under a highway bridge, out of the sunlight. Melted snow had pooled and frozen invisibly. It hadn't even occurred to me that ice might be the problem, or I would have pumped rather than pushed on the brake pedal. No wonder my efforts were futile.

Having an explanation helps, when things go out of control. It helps if you can make sense of what happened. Sometimes things don't make sense at all. I can't help but think of a friend of mine, whose husband simply disappeared one day, having secretly hidden, even from his accountant, his manipulations of his company's finances. His departure left the company in unredeemable ruin and left her with debts that forced her into poverty, after more than twenty years of living an affluent lifestyle with him. It was a devastating severance of trust. She didn't suspect a thing. Everything she had relied on was suddenly, inexplicably gone. It took her years to rebuild her life and her confidence.

I think of another friend who discovered her husband in sexual contact with their three-year-old daughter. She had relied on him, was firmly bound to him as her lifetime partner, and appreciated his exceptionally fine abilities as a parent. Suddenly, what she had counted on was no longer reliable. Her trust was shattered. Her life was in frantic disarray for years afterward.

Trust is a fragile thing. When you can't count on what you could always count on, there is a raw, naked, falling feeling. Like when you lean against something that appears solid, but isn't nailed down, and it gives way. You think you have planted yourself safely, but you have not. I knew this feeling in a very pointed way behind the wheel of my car that day. I had pressed on the brake and my sense of certainty gave way. I was shaken by the experience. All the rest of that afternoon, a shrill, wailing cry was waiting to come out from a hollow, empty space inside me. Yet it remained unheard, despite my being among a sizeable, friendly group of people.

I was with a group of old friends that day, people I used to spend much of my time with when I was married. For more than twenty years, they had been a grounding force, an anchor for me. They were all still married and still spent a lot of time together. But I didn't see much of them anymore. I'd talk with a few of them now and then, but only on rare occasions, such as decade birthdays, would I reconnect with them as a group. This was Anita's fiftieth birthday party, and a large group of people gathered at her house. The first part of the afternoon, it was just the old circle of friends. Later, other guests would arrive, including my former husband.

I was glad to be there, but I felt awkward. I hadn't been on the trips to Mexico these friends had taken together and were discussing. I wasn't up on the series of illnesses some of them had experienced and the job changes and family affairs that were the context for the conversation. I was an outsider, feeling alternate rushes of sadness for what used to be and gladness for being back in this old circle of friends. I became markedly aware of the absence of the closeness I had once felt with them. I knew that I had a different circle of close friends now, yet the edges around the hole in my heart caused by the distance I felt from these old friends were beginning to bleed. I puzzled over why these weren't my closest friends anymore. It wasn't the divorce so much. The parting of ways had started earlier. I still don't exactly know why. The divorce and my moving to another part of town plus the moves of other group members accelerated the dissolution of closeness. It was sad, in a way, yet in my mind I convinced myself it was all right. The past was the past. I could hold our former closeness as a treasure once possessed, now tenderly held in memory. And I could do the dance of today with them comfortably, rediscovering who they were now, if not for closeness, then simply for the fun of it. I could if my heart weren't bleeding.

Someone suggested that, before the evening guests arrived, we could go to the Minneapolis Institute of Arts to see Dale Chihuly's exhibit of blown glass. I was relieved. The tone of conversation had been strangely flat, boring even, and the afternoon had seemed long. I offered to be one of the drivers, and three of the group rode with me. Our efforts at small talk on the way to the museum were just that. The hole seemed to be getting bigger, and I had nothing right then to cover it with or to help stop the bleeding. It was on the way to the museum, while driving with a fragile heart, that the van appeared stationary in front of me, and the brakes didn't hold.

After we got to the museum, group members seemed to pair up easily, and I found myself walking through the exhibit alone. My legs were shaking. My heart was raw. The walls were not solid around me. Nothing seemed familiar, and indeed it wasn't. Chihuly's gigantic, swirling, brilliantly lit glass creations were otherworldy. They made me want to play, to splash paint, to dance. Yet, I was bleeding still and moved slowly. I watched a long video about Chihuly and his colleagues obviously enjoying their collaborative work of quickly, creatively shaping huge bubbles of hot glass amidst loud music. It looked like fun. I wanted to create something big and wild and beautiful like that, something massive enough to express the sweetness of old friendships that never really die and the pain of being unanchored in their midst. I wanted to tell the world I felt powerless, out of control, *unable* to control, unable to trust what I had once trusted in the same way anymore, and that this helpless surrender into empty space was both frightening and freeing and as exquisite as a Chihuly creation, so exotic and yet so vulnerable to being broken.

Returning to Anita's house, I wondered if I should stay. More people were arriving, the food was ready. I decided to eat and hang around awhile longer. The mood of the party was still rather subdued. But, before long, the energy and the volume of conversation seemed to pick up. Maybe it was the critical mass of people; maybe it was Ben's infectious, gregarious greeting and big laugh when he arrived. I was drawn by his smile even after all this time. He sat well away from me, just as he usually did when we were married. We barely glanced at each other as we have come to do. I thought I would be okay with him being there. Even though I was still open-wounded from the afternoon's events, even though it was one of very few times he and I had both been together in a gathering of this old circle of friends, I thought I had enough emotional distance after five years to take his presence there more or less in stride.

I kept distant for a while anyway. But the mix of loss and sweet memories began to permeate the room, like the fragrance of lilacs. When I smell lilacs, the experience is always bitter-sweet, reminding me of the childhood springtimes on the farm, where lilac bushes were huge and abundant. I miss those times, yet savor them. Suddenly, like the van moving too closely into view, I became aware that two of the couples in the room used to be part of a marriage enrichment group Ben and I had belonged to. Anita and Hank and Janine and Bill used to meet monthly with us and a fourth couple, sometimes right in this very living room, to find ways to examine and strengthen our own marriages. These had been tender times, where truth got spoken, obstacles unearthed, encouragement offered. Now, we were in the same room together again. The others were still married. Ben and I were each there alone. Something I had once trusted to be there like a mountain wasn't there anymore. I had recognized this many times before, but each time it showed up in yet another form, in another memory, it jarred me.

Sitting there, I felt my right foot pushing against the floor, with all the strength in my foot, my leg, my middle. Then both feet pressed down. Every muscle in my body strained, right up through my forehead. My entire body was elongated, my bottom raised slightly off the chair where I sat, my shoulders jammed against its back. I generated a surge of strength that felt powerful enough to stop a train. I was giving it all I had. It wasn't enough. There were no brakes as I once again encountered the pain of our separateness. I hadn't seen the ice. My heart crashed defenselessly. There was no sense to be made of it. My body collapsed, weary and wet.

I looked around. Conversations continued; no one had noticed. I rose and walked unsteadily into the kitchen, where one friend who had been my closest was alone, arranging food. "It's kind of weird being here with Ben," I understated, gingerly testing the safety of exposing my wound.

"I suppose," she replied. Her voice was tender, so were her eyes. "It's weird for the rest of us, too. We haven't seen the two of you together that often." She is the one who had informed me in advance, cautiously, that Ben would be there. Even when you know ahead of time and you prepare yourself for reunions such as this, you can't anticipate the ice under the bridge or how your passengers will be affected. And no matter how hard you push, the brakes may not hold.

🌀 Chapter Six

Carrying Weights

ike and I sat on the living room floor facing each other, just as we had done almost every Sunday evening for more than two years. We met to discover whatever we could about our internal lives and to support each other's growing edges. I had gotten to know Mike, a tall, partially bald man with big, kind eyes, at a personal empowerment workshop. We quickly felt a kinship and decided to meet weekly for mutual support. Our evenings together had no agenda. We simply did our best to tune in to what wanted to happen. Always there were shifts and revelations, often quite surprising.

As usual this evening, we began by declaring what was stirring inside us at the moment and reporting on developments of the week. I felt weighted, I told him, five-hundred-pounds thick. Like an enormous crate sunken in a deep, empty well and settled in the darkness with too little air. Every breath felt like hard work, with each inhalation requiring my chest to lift a great many pounds.

Mike's penetrating eyes were at full attention. He waited—minutes—until I could lift my voice enough to say more.

"I sold my piano," I said. "They took it away this week."

The words were dredged up from the well bottom. I could barely speak them. The message sounded mundane, as if I had said it rained again or I washed clothes. I wanted the words to be screamed—*heard*—but my voice, like the rest of me, was deadweighted. I looked to Mike to see if he understood. He did not. How could he? It was my weight. I tried to explain: I had loved this piano for more than three decades. But the words remained dry, boxy, restrained.

⭢

The piano was a Chickering; an upright grand it was called, built in the early 1900s. Very heavy, the movers said. Substantial, I thought. Grand indeed. Worth its weight. It was moved into our house thirty years ago, handpicked by the president of Schmitt Music Company because he was a good friend. All three of us played it: Ben; our son, André; and I.

André, a small-built, tan-skinned boy with his father's handsome looks and a bright disposition, played for the three or four years he took lessons. He learned fast and practiced fast, but his hyper energy made him too impatient for the required daily half-hour of practice. He simply could not play a song over and over until it was smooth. His teacher, a hyper woman herself, understood his high-speed drive, so she didn't make him play through a whole piece very often, just enough to show he had the hang of it. That's the way he practiced, too, just enough to get by. I'd try to sit with him on the bench sometimes and help him with the hard parts. I wanted so badly for him to have the experience of mastering the piano, for all the joy it could bring. But he couldn't seem to still his rapid-fire mind and body, and he'd interrupt me and refuse to go over something more than twice. Once I slapped him as he chattered away and banged on the keys while I was talking. I was markedly startled by my action and struck with immediate remorse. It wasn't the only time his restless energy had tested my patience, but it was the only time I had ever hit him. The piano lessons ended soon after.

The person most faithful to the piano was Ben. With his broad shoulders and his head of close-cut, tightly curled, salt-and-pepper hair bent over the keyboard, he pounded out a few boogie-woogie pieces two or three times a week, but it was "Moonlight Sonata" that he played time and again. He had memorized it, and it soothed him when he felt surly. His playing soothed me, too, the melodic repetitions of the sonata especially. Ben played the piano hard, with a decisive deliberateness. His pure notes and mistruck ones could be heard loudly. He'd replay a phrase, sometimes two or three times, sometimes with pounded irritation, until the right notes were found. Over time, his hard, thick fingernails scraped away at the piano's cherry finish, leaving two half-moon imprints engraved behind the middle C octave.

I, too, played the piano to soothe myself. My playing was quieter, more tentative. My mistakes were frequent, and I felt great embarrassment as I made the corrections or sometimes just slid over the bad notes as if they were intentional. It never felt smooth to me, my playing. I wasn't hyper like André, but like him I wasn't willing to play and play again until I got it right. I wanted to get it right at first sight and was annoyed that I couldn't. Still, I played when it suited me. Even an awkwardly played "Für Elise" or Tchaikovsky's Piano Concerto no. 1 calmed me and gave welcome expression to my passions, most of the time outweighing my self-criticism.

The piano came with me after the divorce. The movers complained of its unusual heaviness. Not surprising. It had absorbed the full weight of our family's fiery forces without being consumed by them. I had tried to sell the piano. Ben had insisted that he should get half of the price even though the divorce settlement was long over. In his mind, that piano wasn't part of the original deal. It wasn't the same as the chairs, the rocker, the table, the couch. This was a personal belonging. It still carried his hard-played songs. Legally, he had no case, but as often happened when we were married, I wasn't able to resist his angered insistence. It also felt like the right thing to do. If he'd had room in his apartment, he'd have taken it when we divorced. I had felt sad at the time that he couldn't, knowing how much it meant to him.

I couldn't find a buyer for the piano readily, and André, who was heartbroken over having to leave the home of his childhood, asked if we could take it with us when we moved. He still played it from time and time. I agreed, realizing that I, too, wanted to bring this part of home with me.

A piano felt like a permanent fixture to me, just as it did in my childhood home. The old upright in our farmhouse sat in the living room all during my childhood, rarely needing tuning. My older sisters had played it when I was growing up, and I took lessons myself for two or three years starting in second grade. Sister Albertine, bone-thin and wrinkled, seemed pleased at how quickly I caught on. My mother was glad to have me playing, even though she would have rather heard a polka than a Concerto in C. She made sure I practiced every day, and I gladly obliged most of the time. I'd loved being able to learn new songs. I imagined that they sounded as grand as I'd heard on the record player. Mom would have me perform for company and she came to all of my recitals. I took great pride in the attention and accolades. My dad didn't want to "listen to that noise" when he came home, because of his headaches. But that never discouraged me.

We couldn't afford lessons after my dad died when I was eight, but Sister Albertine continued them, in part out of sympathy, I suspect, but also because our family had given one of our members to the seminary and one to the convent, and my mother was always helping out at church. We were "good Catholics," and, in effect, I was a charity case for the sisters. But my mother couldn't allow that to go on for more than a year, so I had to quit the lessons. I was sad.

Still, I continued playing throughout my childhood. Summer afternoons I would sit on the piano bench for an hour at a stretch, playing songs in my John W. Schaum lesson books. Those books, plus a few recital pieces, familiarized me with Chopin, Handel, Beethoven, and Mozart. I would spread wide my right thumb and pinkie to pound out the *dum, dum, dum, dum* opening descent of Tchaikovsky's Piano Concerto no. 1. When I did, my youthful passions, stoically contained within my German Catholic upbringing, leaked out onto the keyboard. I felt the might of triumphant marches, the tiptoeing of andante passages, the giddiness of concluding crescendos. There were moments, after the final note of a concerto was struck, that the brief silence was broken, right there in our living room, by the rousing applause and unbridled cheers from an *Ed Sullivan Show* audience. I stood and bowed graciously, acknowledging the world's appreciation. At other times, it was enough for me that my common boredom, loneliness, and disappointments had been absorbed by the piano and transformed into melodic sounds that lifted my spirits.

I wanted very much to play popular music, too, but my fifty-cent weekly allowance only permitted a rare purchase of sheet music, which usually became a disappointment. The plinking of "Don't Be Cruel" on the piano sounded flatly uninteresting against my radio memory of Elvis' seductive singing.

In reality, I was never very good at playing piano, and once I was away at college, where the piano wasn't within easy reach, lack of practice meant diminished skill. Someday I'll get back to the piano, I kept thinking. A few years later, bringing the Chickering into our home excited me. The thrilling and satisfying transformations I remembered from those mighty marches and giddy crescendos would be mine again. Over the years during my marriage, I did play the piano off and on, but in my busy days of working and parenting, I rarely allowed myself much time for this leisurely pleasure. And, without faithful playing, the clumsiness I felt each time I sat down again almost always brought more discouragement than delight. Still, the piano was there. It wasn't the piano of my childhood, but it looked and sounded a lot like that one, and it brought under my roof the memories and possibilities of those long-ago summer afternoons. It also beckoned "someday" to me. It was a place of promise for my passions.

Once moved to my new home after the divorce, the piano became mainly a fixture. André rarely played it before moving out on his own two years later. I sat down to play now and then, but as I spent more and more time working at the computer, the thought of maintaining the same posture at another keyboard during my leisure time had less and less appeal. The fact that the piano sat in my office—the only available space for it—also made it less attractive. Yet there it was, a faithful fixture, and a beautiful piece of furniture at that. Its cherry color burned brightly in the morning sunlight, especially after being touched up with English Leather. It was a hearth, the holder of many fires, some still burning.

One day I mentioned casually to a friend that I should probably get rid of the piano. I hadn't played it in at least three years, and it had gone way out of tune. If I didn't sell it before its value was completely lost in the prevailing small-piano market, I feared I might have to pay to have it taken away. It had also become obvious to me that the "someday" of playing it again would probably not happen, reinforced by a recent diagnosis of arthritis. It was a dream best passed along to someone else, I thought.

My friend immediately told me she knew someone at her workplace in the market for an old upright. Here's my chance, I thought. I can get rid of it without the hassle of advertising. Her friend wanted to see it right away.

The moment I made the decision to sell it, a massive heaviness fell over me. A very low minor chord had been struck and held. It wouldn't let go of me. The days that passed before the movers came, I looked at the piano often. It looked substantial, beautiful, homey. It seemed to belong where it stood, a friend who had taken up a lot of space in my life, the kind with whom long periods in silence were comfortable.

Three men were needed to move it, half the number for a casket. Their big winter boots tracked on the carpet, but they were quick with the job. It was just a big wooden box to get through two doorways and onto a truck. I should have been allowed a few moments to throw dirt into the grave before they finished their job. But they headed off with my piano to the home of Leeann and Will and their eager little boy, Thatcher. He had been asking Leeann every day when it was coming, and Leeann wanted to study piano, too, she told me, but mostly she just wanted a piano in her home, right in the living room. Yes, that's where it belonged.

During our time together on Sunday evenings, Mike and I sometimes sat for periods in silence—honoring what had gone before or awaiting with curious anticipation what might come forth next from one of us. After I told him of the great weight harbored within my body, stillness settled around us as if concert hall lights had just dimmed and the curtain was rising. At last, the big wooden box with tight strings and dusty insides, which was gone after being silent for so long, yet which now resided as a heavy weight encompassing me, could no longer hold back its song. Moist music—its music—seeped out of me in a long keening over lost dreams, replaying sweet and sour love notes, mourning the never-reached crescendo of someday. Mike sat with me and listened for a half hour or more until my piano's farewell song came to its end.

That piano had been a bedrock for me. As long as its hefty presence, embedded with its passionate memories, was there, I had felt close to the ground, secure. Even after my husband and son were gone, I had counted on the piano and all that it held to keep me company.

"I don't have a lot to anchor me these days," I said to Mike.

"I know. Sometimes I think I've been an anchor for you."

"Yes. You. And the piano. And a few others who stay with me."

I remember when a friend told me his grandfather had died. He said he would miss his gentle ways, his laughter. My friend said that in order to keep those cherished qualities of his grandfather alive, he would have to assume them for himself. I told this story to Mike. After another period of silence, I rose to my feet. Softened by long-sobbed sounds, I felt the timber of the cherry wood slowly melding with my bones and sinew. The moisture had made it live, supple. The weight no longer felt leaden but planted. I began to sway. I felt as if dead branches began to fall away, and new roots descend. Reaching my arms upward, I sang a clear, loud, sustained low note and stood tall and steady.

Part Two

Lies My Mother Told Me

The horizon, to our eyes, appears flat. Deception clouds perception. What don't we know that we don't know?

Slow Down the Hurry Up

*A*n exercise I sometimes use in the Writing Your Own Permission Slip course is having participants complete the sentence fragment, "My mother always said . . ." Since I do the exercise myself each time as well, my litany of remembered maternal commands, demands, and moral advisories has been growing quite long: *Be careful. Behave yourself. Say your prayers. Do what you're told. What's the matter with you kids; can't you get anything right? You should be ashamed of yourself. What will people think? Don't be so silly.* As the youngest of nine children, I heard these same messages frequently reiterated by older siblings as well.

These directives were said with vehemence, and often with some level of threat implied. They were not to be taken lightly, and I didn't. I became careful, well-behaved, obedient. I said my prayers. I was ashamed of myself a lot. I worried about what people thought. I took on the cloak of seriousness. In fact, I became annoyingly rigid and preachy as a child, prompting other kids to keep their distance.

One of my mother's directives that I remember most emphatically was, Hurry up! *Hurry up and eat your breakfast, or you'll be late for school. Hurry up and get in the car, or we'll be late for church. Hurry up or I'll give you a reason to hurry up. Get in here this minute or else . . .* In each of these admonitions, there was always the *or else* implied if not spoken. I complied because I didn't want to risk a certain scolding or a slap with the ruler or at least the inevitable shame

I'd feel for failing to get things done, for being late, for not getting something *right*—and in a hurry.

My mother wasn't a particularly mean person. In fact, her pleasantly plump face and figure and her come-on-over-for-dinner-anytime way of treating people exuded a mother-hen kindness that kept visitors sitting long at our table. Yet, there was also a rigid sternness about her also that demanded hurry, perfection, and punctuality from her children. Where this sternness came from, I can't exactly say. Maybe keeping up with the needs of nine children wore out her patience and energy. Maybe she adopted this way of operating from her own mother. Maybe it emerged from our Germanic or Catholic traditions. One thing was clear: there was one right way to do things, and I'd better do it—fast. These influences led me to a life often propelled by righteousness, expediency, and compulsion in an effort to please (whomever was nearby) through disciplined, high-speed accomplishment. I was the first one with a hand up in class and the first to get done when a test was given. I raced to school in the morning, arriving early so I could offer (quick) help before class and become the teacher's pet. Later, in my early fifties, I raced through graduate school, often enduring high stress and exhaustion rather than heeding my advisor's counsel to slow down and enjoy the process. I was still living out the story created from my mother's directives embedded in my psyche and in every cell of my body since infancy.

That's the story I tell about how I was raised—part of it, at least. For each of us, what we say about our experience is just that—a story. It's not what *actually* happened, but rather the way we choose to describe our life. In creating our story, we select certain things to include and leave out others. We create good guys and bad guys. We decide if our stories are comedies or tragedies. Over time, we develop core stories or myths that answer the big questions about who we are, where we came from, why we're here, what we're to do, what constitutes success, and what will happen after death. Our stories define us. We become the stories that we tell ourselves. They literally shape us emotionally and physically. They are our identity, and we can't do anything in our lives beyond what our self-defining stories allow. Roger Schank, a scholar of personal narrative, sums this up nicely in *Tell Me a Story: Narrative and Intelligence* by saying, "We are the stories we like to tell." He says that as we tell our stories over and over, "these stories become who we are and telling them allows us to feel these feelings that define us yet again."

Our bodies express these stories, even if they are never spoken aloud. We *feel* them, and we're shaped by them. If we're told to shut up a lot as a kid, we may create a story about having nothing to say and gradually tighten our vocal muscles. If we're scared a lot, we may create a story about being in danger or having to be brave, and walk around with our chests caved in for protection or stuck out in defiance or feigned courage. A woman told me she got diabetes when she was eleven, and years later, when a therapist asked her if anything significant had happened around the time the diabetes started, she said that her brother was born, the boy her father had always wanted. Until then, she had been her father's treasure. "The sweetness went out of your life," the therapist said, offering a possible explanation for her illness. The woman nodded.

Adult stories, as well as childhood ones, leave an imprint on our bodies. Ted, a friend of mine, once owned a large, flourishing printing company and lived a show-off life, throwing cash freely at airplanes, boats, cars, and travel. He liked to impress friends and clients with the ability to fly them anywhere they wanted in his own plane. After a heart attack, a messy divorce, bankruptcy, and a series of other problems with family, finances, and health, Ted became weighted down with depression. That was about twenty years ago. Since then, Ted has gotten counseling and reassessed his priorities. Now, in his sixties, he lives on a bare-survival income, and his main interest is in cultivating unpretentious, intimate friendships. But his body has not forgotten the old story of glory.

One day Ted excitedly took the seven-year-old "little brother" he was mentoring to a small airport's open house. Ted was thrilled to show the boy the various planes and equipment on display and tell him how everything worked. The boy was enthralled. But Ted found himself feeling strangely disheartened and drained on the way home afterward. Soon, he had severe diarrhea. The next day, Ted told me, "I couldn't figure out where this came from out of the blue, why I was feeling so emotional and why I had this diarrhea. But I finally figured it out. Being back at the airport where I had spent so much time when I had a lot of money, I realized how much I missed all those fun times—being able to do whatever I wanted, to fly wherever I wanted to go. I remembered all the things that had gotten me into such trouble, how full of shit I was." Then, seeing the irony, he laughed and said, "No wonder I got diarrhea! I guess I'm still trying to get rid of all that crap."

In his book *The Healing Power of Stories*, Daniel Taylor confirms that our old, painful stories tend to stay with us as a corrosive force, like street salt rusting away a car's frame. He says, "We cling even to broken stories precisely because they are the only stories we know, or the only ones we can imagine ourselves living. It feels safer to accept the pain with which we are familiar than to risk the unknown pain that may be a part of change." But he also says, "New stories lead to new actions, and new actions to new stories."

Ted continues to work at changing the story he lived by for so long, through noticing the emotions behind his bodily reactions to situations and drawing on the support of friends. Sometimes it takes many years, but stories can get revised and retold when we're ready. That's the main premise of my Permission Slip class in which people let their bodies reveal and revise self-limiting scripts and update promising ones that have been dormant. It's also what I watch happening over and over again in my own life and with friends like Ted.

Shortly after I turned fifty, I decided to take a sabbatical. Right on schedule with midlife's normal impetus to self-reflection and redirection, I felt an urgent, compelling desire to *slow my life way down* and explore something I couldn't yet define. My budget didn't allow me to take a sabbatical in the usual sense of going away for an extended period of time to study something of interest. But, I decided I could take another type of "leave," a sabbatical from everything but the most essential work I needed to do to make my living. I cut way back on social and service activities that packed every work-free hour of my schedule. Then, I became very quiet for a few months. I spent the bulk of my time alone, rarely made phone calls, and listened only to the sounds of nature and the necessary kitchen and computer noises as I handled daily tasks. TV, radio, and even my tape player were mostly silent. Staring out the window for hours and taking nature walks became favorite pastimes.

Much like sports replays done in slow motion, this process of slowing myself way down let me observe pivotal moves (mental and physical) that led toward either satisfying or not-so-satisfying results in my life. I had long known that there are precise moments when our thoughts take a turn toward trouble and that there are corresponding warning signals in our bodies. Now, in my slowed-down mode, I could actually observe these phenomena reflectively, without rushing.

One of my discoveries was that my usual *first thought* and corresponding *first move* were to rush, rush, rush. Mind and body were living the "hurry up" story of childhood. This was no small matter for me, as it had led to many years of agonizing and disabling panic attacks, complete with sudden, terrifying symptoms of rapid heartbeat, shortness of breath, feeling faint, mental disorientation, irritability, and more.

Now, operating in slow-motion mode, I noticed the exact moment in a situation when I began introducing a "hurry up" message and a corresponding "or else." I could feel when my body began pumping out adrenaline in sync with the panicky thoughts. With my now uncrowded calendar, I had the time to gently, gradually reorient my thinking to a no-need-to-rush mode. I could observe my "hurry up" thoughts and let them pass through. I could try different ones.

Though I was operating in a leisurely manner during my non-work hours in this sabbath period, I was often still driven by my "hurry up" story in my work life. One client, with whom I was developing a huge curriculum, was a brilliant, wildly creative, and ambitious man. Every time we spoke, he'd have another remarkable new idea about how to reorganize or expand the project. I was intrigued by his quick mind, his broad knowledge and superb memory, and his knack for frequent complex re-envisioning and expanding of the project, but our conversations often left me in a spin. I'd put down the phone after talking with him and massive self-doubt would set in. Tension in my neck and shoulders, low back pain, and a nervous stomach quickly recorded the aftermath.

One day I slowed down enough to observe these reactions more closely, and a familiar litany of thoughts rolled across my mental screen. I jotted them down in my journal:

> I feel so out of control on this project, like I never know what will happen, like I'll never get it figured out. I feel so insecure—afraid I won't be able to keep up, won't remember, won't get done in time, won't know what to do, will look foolish, and will be thought badly of.

My array of feelings and thoughts reminded me of an experience I had when I was about ten years old. My mother sent me to the basement, where she kept a supply of canned goods, to get a jar of beets. Though I looked and looked, I couldn't find any beets on the shelves. I remember the panic and shame I felt—what a failure that meant I was. *I can't figure this out. I don't know what to do. She's going to be so mad if I don't hurry up and find them.* My neck and my belly tensed, my breathing became shallow, my eyes darted about, desperate to accomplish my mission before Mom would start to holler at me. I remember walking up the stairs, with my head low and shoulders rounded, already somatically shaped by the anticipated scolding.

I continued writing in my journal, this time rewriting the story that had me by the neck. I began with, "I know the truth about myself," and then created a new nonmaternal litany to try out, "I am doing the best I can. There is no right way to do this. It's okay if I don't always look good. Even if I come up short or people don't like me, I'm still all right. I'll find a way to handle whatever happens." I concluded with, "There is no rush. Everything will get done in due time." As I wrote each sentence, I tried to breathe it into my bones. I wanted to believe it, to experience it, to have it take hold. I wanted it as a new chapter heading in my story. I also knew that writing it on paper was only a first step. The real change would happen as I revised the story I was living in my outlook and actions day by day.

When I imagined living as if I believed that everything would get done in due time, without rushing, and as if other people's opinions of me were no longer a standard for judging myself, these notions seemed both as appealing and as hard to achieve as my client's visions. Yet my new written litany warmed me to the possibility. *What if? What if I could live like that?*

I wanted the change to happen immediately, of course. After all, I had a mind and body well-trained in hurry-up mode, so a story revision like this seemed like it shouldn't take all that long. But first-draft versions emerging from early life experiences can seem too familiar and comfortable to give up easily. "Change the thought, change your life," the motivational speakers say. "Just do it." But, hearing that, my speed-conditioned psyche jumps to: *I'd better get better right now, or else.* How insidious are the lies that sear our minds and bodies, burning sagas of deception into every corner of the cortex, into every ligament and tendon, even into every heartbeat. I know that miraculous healing of the body sometimes happens, and I suppose, by the same token, our internal story revisions can sometimes be instantaneous. But more often, many drafts are what make a fine manuscript.

The next three chapters reveal some of my revision process during the early, middle, and more recent stages of restorying my life. All along the way, my body has been a principal character in the changing story—telling of the tension between holding on to the old and opening up to the new. The story revisions are unfinished, of course. They will continue over time as my body tugs at me to play it safe even while pressing for the freedom to play it real.

🌀 Chapter Eight

The Silent Sanctuaries of Shame

*I*n the name of the Father and the Son and the Holy Ghost. I can reach the holy water fountain real easy now that I'm nine. The cool water on my forehead makes me shiver. I'm already cold from walking the six blocks to St. Catherine's. I come here almost every Saturday for confession. I want to be good, like the sisters say. St. Catherine's is big inside, so big that I would have to stack a hundred of me on top of each other to touch the ceiling. And it's dark in here, because the sun isn't shining. When it's sunny, the saint pictures on the stained glass windows make the church so pretty with green and blue and yellow just like in my paint set. It's quiet in here, the way it always is on Saturdays. *Oh no! My footsteps click way too loud.* "Shhh! Don't be so noisy!" That's what my mom would say. Everyone is probably looking at me, or trying not to. I look down. I'm embarrassed, but I try to look pious so everyone will see I'm sorry for disturbing them. From now on, I'll tiptoe.

Power on. Start belt. I step onto the treadmill's black moving surface attentively, adjusting quickly to its speed. The gauge reads 1.2 miles per hour. I quickly urge it upward to 2.4, 3.0, 3.5, 3.6. No, too fast. 3.5. That's better. I don't feel like pushing it today. I have made myself come here, but the weightiness inside my chest and belly adds resistance. I've felt heavy, stuck, all day. That's been going on for a while now, this icky sense of being a mistake. It really hit me hard today, over nothing really. I settle in, legs coaxed into automatic momentum, arms swinging alternately in sync. Mind quickly slipping into neutral, shutting out the day.

I tiptoe to a pew about halfway down the aisle. When I genuflect, I almost lose my balance. I've been so clumsy lately. Mom says it's because I got a whole inch taller since last year and I don't know what to do with it. But I've always been kind of clumsy. That's why I never get chosen 'til last when kids pick sides for kickball. I trip all the time. After I get in the pew and kneel down, I lean back to take off my jacket, but I shiver, so I put it back on. This place is so cold. *Lookit! There's Jim Thilmony coming in the other end of my pew in shirtsleeves! He should have a coat on.* He's the most handsome basketball player for St. Catherine's, with his wavy brown hair and football shoulders. The high school girls giggle a lot around him. I'll bet they don't know he's my brother's friend and he comes over to *my* house *all the time.* I adjust the hanky on top of my head, straighten my dress, and show my dimples a little. He does not notice me.

I look at the clock. It is 4:47. Five to ten minutes of warm-up on the treadmill, the trainer advised. The high-speed fan in front of me blows too-cool air. Noticing the man on the next treadmill jogging aggressively and perspiring, I swing my arms with more vigor. I glance at the other people on treadmills. They are all moving forward, looking forward, unaware of me. Most wear headphones. I am shut out. It used to be like that in church when I was a kid—everyone looking straight ahead, no one talking. *Who knows, maybe some of these people are saying their prayers. Maybe I should say some.* I look at the bikers and stair climbers facing me. Eyes meet for only the second it takes to not recognize someone and move on.

The line at each confessional is long. There are maybe eight to ten people in each one. I look to see if any of my friends are there, but they aren't. *They should come here every Saturday like I do, so they don't go to hell.* I see Mrs. Beckerleg. I call her the pumpkin lady because she's so round. She's always smiling when I meet her, but now she's not. I wonder if it was a mortal sin when she kicked out her husband. I would never do that. Theresa is in line, too. She's in high school and she's kind of shy. Her skirt is too long and her sweater has those little balls on it. Her clothes look old like mine, hand-me-downs. I walk to school with her sometimes, and she seems interested even when I talk too much. I wonder what her sins are.

From time to time, people walk in. Their eyes scan the all-occupied treadmills. Only one man stops. He stands, leaning against the wall with his arms folded, waiting. He is muscular, lean, with a well-carved dimple along his angular chin. My age. I look at his left hand. No ring. I stand taller, smile a little. He is gazing at the ceiling. After a while, my smile fades. *Maybe if I were thinner, wore nail polish, knew how to roll my curves just right as I walk . . .* Of the twenty or so people in the room, only two people are talking to each other, a young woman and an elderly man on adjoining stationary bikes. They chat eagerly, laughing from time to time, but thankfully I hear only edges of their exchange over the rumbling and whirring of the machines. *If he had even looked my way, acknowledged I'm here . . . , but why would he, the way I look?*

A fidgety girl drops her rosary on the floor. The beads rattle as they strike the floor. She lifts the kneeler so she can reach the rosary, and the kneeler clunks loudly. Some people look at her. Her face gets red and she is real careful not to make a sound when she lowers the kneeler to the floor. *She should be more careful.* From time to time, I hear whispers from the confessional of sins being told. Father Dawson's whispers are louder as he gives the penance. Sometimes the confession takes a long time. I try to hear, and try not to hear. *What is taking so long?* At last, the little sliding door clacks shut. The person is finished. A few eyes turn to see who's coming out. *What was their sin? What penance has Father given them?* Meantime the door has slid open on the other side so Father can hear the next person already in place.

Steady pace. Breathing harder. Step, step, step, step, step, step. Three minutes, twenty seconds. No one's talking now. A bare-shouldered teenager sashays through the door of the tanning room. *Nothing on this body to apologize for. Maybe those hips have done some things. She has not learned to brush her long hair over her shoulder just to impress herself. What a shame girls that young are so sex-crazed. But, god, I'd like to look that good.* Step, step, step, step, more of me in motion now. The window to the aerobics room reflects my full-tummy outline, the glint of my glasses, the same old haircut. Clock hand creeps.

I sit down and take a look at my watch. 3:30. I'm not ready to get in line yet. I have to think of my sins. *What will I say? I argued with Mary Ann yesterday and then Mom yelled at us. Let's see. Did I disobey Mom? No, when she yelled at me, I stopped talking, like she said. Was I mean to Mary Ann? Yeah, I guess I was mean. Okay, there's one sin, I was mean to my sister once. I told Mom she was the one who started it. Maybe that was a lie. Well, she did start it because she was the one who*

told me to get over on my own side of the bed. I wasn't that far on her side, maybe an inch, that's all. I got so mad at her! She just wanted to pick on me about something, that's all. No, I didn't start it. I didn't lie about that. But I shouldn't have said she pushed me first though. She didn't. I was the one who pushed. Jesus wouldn't like that. Okay, I lied once. I hang my head and fold my hands, but my jaws are pushed together because I'm still thinking about what Mary Ann said. That's all the sins I can think of. I look at the lines by the confessional and pick the shorter one. But then I change my mind. *I'm sure I forgot something. I must be more sinful than that.* I decide to do the stations of the cross to work up some feelings of guilt.

Five minutes to go. *I really screwed up today. Marlys gave me a big compliment, and what did I do? Oh, I really don't want to think about it. I'll just keep my eye on the clock, it's almost time to go to the Nautilus room. I can't believe how stupid my response was. Here I was, called into an important meeting in an executive conference room. Marlys had picked me to bring in as the expert. She even said that both she and the director of the organization thought of me at the same time as the perfect person for the job. So, fine, leave it at that. Just remember she has lots of faith in you. Don't even think about how you said such a dumb thing. It's no big deal. But what was I doing in a place like that, with people of that caliber! Surely, it was a mistake that I was there.* Lord, I am not worthy. *At least lately, I haven't been able to do anything right.*

That's what it feels like anyway. There's a pervasive glumness in my chest, and I walk around with stooped shoulders. I must be doing things wrong, or I'd be getting more people calling on me, wanting my services. I must be out of touch, behind the times. Someone must have found out that though I look very competent, put on a good show, I'm just bluffing. I don't really know what I'm doing most of the time.

I felt totally inept in that meeting. I couldn't think of one intelligent thing to say. Well, I did talk, too much, and I'm sure they thought I was way too know-it-all. Then, afterward, when Marlys gave me her usual bright smile and vote of confidence, did I say, "Thank you. I appreciate your faith in me"? No, instead, I had to go and say, "Oh, I suppose I can fumble along 'til I figure it out." Boy, I haven't done that kind of false humility talk in a long time. I feel so foolish. It just came out of nowhere.

The first station, Jesus is condemned to death. Jesus is shown standing before Pilate in the little carving on the wall. He's been beaten and his hands are tied. *He is doing this for me, that's what Sister Rita said. I must be really bad. I must not be saying enough rosaries and studying as much as I should. It's my fault. I try to cry, but no tears come. But I promise to stay with him, even if others hate him. I will try real hard to be good enough, so he doesn't have to go through this.*

Forget about the whole thing. Marlys didn't make a big deal of what I said; why should I? Just keep walking. Seven minutes. Getting a little bored with the pace, even though my energy is picking up. Warm but not perspiring. The runner next to me drips. I judge myself lazy by comparison. *I should be able to run like that. I always give up too easily. If I'd just try harder . . .* My energy drops. The next minute seems eternal. Enough of this. Slow the belt to 3.4, 3.0, 2.4, 2.0. With careful attention, I lift one foot, then the other, and place them on each side of the belt. Press the stop-belt button. Watch until the belt stops moving. Step down onto the nonmoving floor and allow the momentum to shift. Off-balance for just a moment. On to the weight machines downstairs.

I stay with Jesus at the first station until my knees start to feel sore against the hard floor. I stand up—too quickly. I lose my balance. My left ankle twists and shoots out a pin-prick pain. I glance quickly around the church, then duck my head, embarrassed, even though no one's looking. I move on to the other stations, limping more than a little, wincing even though the pain has passed. Maybe if it looks like I'm hurting a lot, people will think it's not from being clumsy, but because I was holy enough to stay kneeling so long. I try to make the pain come back so I don't have to pretend. I hope someone comes over to see if I'm all right. No one notices.

I begin my routine in the exercise room. Ankles first. I sit down and position the balls of my feet on the bars below and then lower the weighted white bar above onto my knees. Lift the knees, drop them slowly. Up, down, up, down, twelve times, each time the strain increases. The last two demand more than I want to give. Next, the hamstring muscles. This time I lift my calves onto padded surfaces and push them down and back under me. Add another five pounds today? No, I just can't. *I suppose I can fumble along.* Push, release, push, release. Eight, nine, ten. This is hard. I stop for a moment. *All right, eleven, yes, twelve.* I stand up, lift the weights to put them away. One slips a little from my hand, tugging a little too hard at an overworked shoulder. I cringe momentarily, look around to see if anyone has noticed, and continue on. Everything seems to hurt today.

Next station. Jesus has already been scourged and crowned with thorns. His clothes are ripped. He is bloody. Now, on top of that, he has to carry a heavy cross. I remember being sharply pricked sometimes as I climbed over barbed wire fences on the farm, and getting rips in my pants. I try to imagine thorns poking into my head and then being made to carry a big cross, too. *How could people be so cruel?* I remember that my mistakes are the thorns and the cross. I put on a sad face and tell Jesus I'm sorry. I promise I will suffer in silence, as he is doing, whenever people are mean to me.

I pick up two ten-pound weights, one in each hand. I hold them at my sides, then shrug and drop my shoulders a dozen times. I continue with several other weights, moving in various positions to strengthen different muscles. I put my right knee on a bench, lean forward a little, and straighten and bend my right arm holding a weight. I remember when I could only lift half as much, and I am satisfied, until I see the tank-topped teenager with long, shiny blond hair next to me raise twenty-five pounds overhead easily. In front of me is a wall covered with mirrors. My graying hair and my eyes sallowed by harsh overhead lights catch my attention, and I notice for the umpteenth time that my jeans and red turtleneck are not standard uniform here. Black and blue spandex is. A dozen or more people glisten in it as they push and grimace and sweat around me. *Where do people buy this stuff? Why am I always so out of fashion?* In some ways, I don't care. Most of the time I don't. I wear what I like, and what I find inexpensively. Today I don't want to run into anyone who knows me, who would see me like this.

I genuflect at the next station and look at the carving there. I try again to cry, scrunching up my face, curling my lower lip, sniffling, but no tears come. *I will try harder to be good, Lord. I won't get mad at my sister. I'll work hard to get all A's. I'll obey Mom all the time. I'll say two rosaries a day.* A side door of the church opens and Sister Rita enters. Even though she has on her long black habit and veil, I recognize her. She is thin and tall like a ghost and she has a stiff walk. She was my teacher last year. She was strict. I obeyed her *all* the time. She does not look around but goes directly to the vigil lights. They are arranged in rows on a large, wrought-iron stand in front of the statue of Mary. I try to catch her eye. I want her to see me making the stations, I want her approving smile for coming to the church by myself and doing the stations on a Saturday. But I know it's not proper to distract her or to show off. I continue with the stations, stiffening a little to be like her. Sisters are probably all saints.

There are at least a dozen people straining around me and moving from machine to machine in silent ritual. A man my height and of trim build, who always wears an orange sweatband, goes through his routines slowly, with care. He glances toward me occasionally, and I toward him. But our eyes never lock. I wonder about him. If I should ever meet him at a social or professional function, we would greet each other with familiarity. *Oh, I always see you at the club.* And we would spend time comparing notes on what all we do here. But, the sanctuarial silence inhibits us now. We remain strangers even though we have both come to this shrine in search of the body's purification. Though we congregate, we abide by the rituals of individual salvation. There is no expressed body of Christ here. We retreat into silence and each carry our own sins, doubts, and desires of body and soul with us from machine to machine, seeking to work out, reduce, firm up what is loose. We do the disciplines of body redemption, and we find our resurrection here. I wonder if he has ever said something stupid.

I jump, startled as Mrs. Beckerleg taps me on the shoulder. She is whispering and has a kind look. "How is your mother ?" I look away, my face gets warm, my tummy queasy. I don't know what to say. When Mom came home from the hospital after Daddy's funeral, she said I shouldn't talk about it. *It's nobody's business.* I didn't know what to say anyway. Mom used to be mad at Dad a lot, so I was surprised she felt bad when he died. She cried a lot, but I didn't. I suppose I should have. I should miss him, too, but I don't especially. Dad was never in the house very much. Even when he was, he was awfully quiet and slept a lot. All I know is, after he died, lots of people came around and gave me lots of attention and even some presents. But Mom went to the hospital. I didn't know why. Now she was home and I was glad.

"Fine," I say to Mrs. Beckerleg. A smile, a pat on the shoulder, and I am left alone again. Her pity settles over me like warm rain through the shoulder she touched. I look to the figure of Jesus on the wall. My mother knows what it means to suffer. At least Father Dawson had a funeral for Daddy and let him be buried in the Catholic cemetery, even though suicide is a mortal sin. Mom was so upset she had to go in the hospital afterward, even though she was sure he couldn't have done it. *He didn't like guns. He didn't even like needles. Every time he had to get a shot, he'd pass out.* She sure cried the night we got the news. *I can't believe I was that terrible to him. Was I that bad a wife?* I'll say these stations for her, so she will get better faster. At the next one, I work up some tears.

⤳

"Hi, how ARE you?" It's Betty, from my old neighborhood, crashing through the silence. "I didn't know you came here." She speaks loudly. Several heads turn our way. I try to quiet her down by speaking softly. *Doesn't she know where she is?* No one speaks here but in low tones. *Shhh!* I tell her I'm fine, that my back pain is much better since I've been coming here. "Great! Nice to see you," she says, then brushes on by me and heads for the bench press. I quickly survey the room. No one is looking now. I'm relieved, then feel foolish. I thought I'd given up my constant opinion charting long ago, too. What does it matter? *What does it matter?*

At the other end of the room, two teenage girls are giggling a little as they try to lift a hundred-pound weight together and can't. *Lighten up. This is supposed to be fun! Give yourself a break. Who cares what people think! Besides, it was nice to connect with Betty, to talk with someone. So what if she broke the rules? I could learn a few things from her. I'll be she wouldn't think what I did today was all that bad.*

She'd just laugh and say, "I've done the same thing myself. Forget it! You're fine!" I mount the low back machine. *Another five pounds today? Hmm . . . Yes! Just watch me.* I clang the weights into place. If someone looks to see who is being so noisy, I don't care.

The seventh station. Jesus falls for the second time. I try to imagine how heavy his cross is. I allow strain to appear on my face. I tell Jesus how sorry I am. I tell him I would have helped if I had been there. I would help Mom, too, if I knew how. I breathe a little harder, my shoulders tense. By the time I get to the ninth station, where Jesus falls for the third time, I feel a pool of warmth growing around my heart and a little wetness in my eyes. I stay on my knees for a long while even though they hurt.

I'm at my last of a dozen stops, the new Gravitron machine. I kneel in the grooves, grasp the bars overhead and lift myself up and down. It's an easy sliding, almost floating sensation as I rise and drop. The arm and back muscles work; but this is pleasure, not penance. Breathe in, breathe out. Easy. I've had whole days like this. I remember now. *Dear God, it's old weight, this being so hard on myself, this shame about everything I do. I thought I'd trimmed that off, lost it for good, but it comes back, it inches up on me.* Just let it flow, easy, up, down, up, down, no strain, no way to do it wrong. *So, I brushed off Marlys' compliment. So what? An old habit came back for a visit, that's all. But, a sign I've gotten careless. That's my sin, God, I got careless. I forgot I am your temple—no less than that. If you have your home in me, can I be so bad? If you live here, I never have to be alone with any of this, I never have to worry if I got it right.*

When I reach the station where Jesus is nailed to the cross, I drop on my knees. I know now I am a sinner. *Look what my sins*

have done. I remember now, I lied three times this week, I was mean once, and I forgot to say my prayers. I step right into line at the confessional. I wait only a minute or so and go in. I am nervous. The air is stale, a blend of cologne and cigarette breath and underarm odor. "Bless me, Father, for I have sinned." I whisper my sins and Father gives me a penance of three Our Fathers and three Hail Marys, as always. I wonder if it would be more if I had sinned more. For a moment, I wonder how I could get him to *talk* to me, to *listen* to me. But I just say, "Thank you, Father." I step out into air where the only smell is candle wax. No one is looking, and I'm glad. Eyes downcast, I kneel once again in a pew and say my penance. I've done what I've been told to do to free myself from my sins. I feel satisfied, sort of, but I wonder if I did it right, if I forgot anything. I rise, genuflect, and turn to leave. I look for someone's nod of approval. No one looks my way. My footsteps click loudly again. *Oh, I forgot.* I cringe in embarrassment and hurry out on my tiptoes.

Now, to the mats. Stretch to the right and hold, and to the left. Lift, down, lift, down. And again, stretch and hold twenty seconds. I know what I need to do for Marlys. It's not that difficult. Just like she said, I'm very capable of doing this work. I'm good at it. I *can* figure it out. What I don't know I can find out. No sweat. *Lord, I know you never look down on me. Help me to remember, to see myself only through your loving eyes.* The fan blows the sweaty smell of a husky man my way. A trainer squats beside him on the next mat. "Hold that position a little longer." I hold mine longer than usual, feeling strong. "That's it. Good workout. Nice going." I feel refreshed, satisfied, redeemed. I look for someone to smile at. No one is available. I smile anyway and take my temple home.

Panic

"*I* can't walk any further," I said reluctantly to my friend Brian, just after we started a short walk before a Sunday morning church service. I had hoped the anxiety of the morning would subside as we got absorbed in conversation, but, typical of my panic attacks, this one was not going to be set aside so easily.

It had started shortly after I woke up and realized this was going to be to an uncluttered day. No work to be done and no plans beyond the church service except a walk with Brian and an evening group meeting. Hours of afternoon free time awaited me. Presumably, this should have been pleasurable. But for me this change from a week of constant activity felt like a sinkhole into which I had stepped unaware. A fall into a vacuum without duty. Unpredictable, without form. My whole system is trained to hurry up, but suddenly there was nothing to hurry for. It made sense then that my heart sped up, that I gasped for air and felt lightheaded. I was in danger of *or else*.

Panic comes on me like that. A thought. Some tiny threat to my safety or security, and it's like being thrown off a ledge. My rationality should save me, but it doesn't. I don't know why exactly. My built-in balancing system, which can assess a threat and determine an appropriate response, has become overly fragile. What should set off a minor alarm triggers a horn blast that sounds a few inches away. My whole system reacts as if a speeding sports car has run a red light just as I enter an intersection.

Racing heart. Shortness of breath. Rushes of heat and cold. Dizzying thoughts. Weakness. Fury mixed with fear. Terror. Panic. Then enormous shame for spinning into this craziness.

I am stopped, unable to take anything but survival actions.

It's been like this for more than twenty years. Sometimes the provocation for the attacks is blatant. Someone yells at me. A critical deadline seems unreachable. Or someone runs a red light just as I enter an intersection. But more often the provoking incident is simply a thought of, well, panic. It can be as simple as realizing I have no planned schedule and suddenly feeling lost, or as monumental as the gripping fear that I will fail at some critical task.

When I catch the triggering thought early enough, I can sometimes redirect it or calm myself by slowing my breathing or imagining a comforting scene. Other times I simply observe the thought ("There must be something I should hurry up for") and the feeling (fear of danger, an adrenaline rush) and recognize that they are just a thought and a feeling which I need not try to change. If the fear and the physical sensations are intense, I have to stop or slow down whatever I'm doing to allow the storm to pass in its own rhythm. I've learned, over time, that though it can feel at its worst as if I will surely pass out or have a heart attack, the feelings will eventually subside. It's not unlike having the flu. I feel awful, and it's hard to function while this condition is at its peak, but I know I'll get better in time, and I just have to be patient with it while it lasts.

I have tried many methods of overcoming these attacks. Medication, support groups, books, meditative practices, therapy, journaling, reasoning, bodywork, homeopathics, acupuncture, qigong, and much more. They've all helped. But the panic attacks continue. Not very often anymore. Not as long-lasting. Not as frightening. But anytime, anyplace, panic can pay me a visit.

I've also learned that I'm not alone in this. Three percent of the population experiences panic attacks. Many suffer in silence.

Most, at some time, probably feel like they're going crazy. Some become depressed. Some lose confidence, jobs, spouses, and other valuables because of these debilitating attacks that come without warning. Many of those I've spoken with have times when they feel great shame and despair at having these bizarre experiences and not being able to stop them. Some *have* been able to stop them, each in their own way. I'm envious. I'm hopeful.

The first time I had one, I was in my thirties. It was a Saturday afternoon and I was heading up a painting party for an inner-city arts education program where I worked. We were refurbishing an old library building and had invited volunteers to spend the afternoon painting walls. A lot was at stake, and I was hyped. We needed lots of people to show up in order do the job. I also wanted to impress a reporter, who was coming from the main metropolitan newspaper, with the amount of community support for this effort. I was on a high-energy roll and was looking for a fast-paced, high-energy crowd eager to paint and have fun together. My own two-year-old and his playmate were there with me, full of energy. They required a constant eye, not only to keep them from running around squealing loudly, but also to keep them safe amidst the construction materials and paint.

Expectations. Mine are too often excessive and too critical for my contentment. I picture how it needs to be and then am driven toward that, determined, assuming it will be so, *must* be so.

Crowds did not come. A few volunteers trickled in, more interested in leisurely chitchat than in my vigorous painting agenda. I was mentally checking the list of all those who hadn't come—friends especially, creating judgments about their absence or conjuring up scenarios about why they might be late and hoping they might still come. I often dashed to the front door to look out and see if anyone else was coming.

Meantime, I was putting brushes in the hands of the two-year-olds who seemed to love splashing yellow onto the walls. I wanted to keep the paint out of their hair and off their shoes—a misplaced expectation. When the reporter came, the children made good photo subjects, but I felt guilty knowing they weren't really "community volunteers." I put on a happy face for my brief interview with him, the same face I'd been showing to the people who had come that afternoon, a face that was half-lying.

As the afternoon progressed, I noticed an occasional heartbeat speed-up. More hoped-for volunteers did not arrive and earlier ones left. Most of the essential-to-paint walls remained untouched. My son and his friend tired and whined and ran squealing. I painted furiously. My shoulders ached. My bad back nagged. The speeding heartbeats made me put the paint roller down for a few minutes. Food might help, I thought. I always think food might help. But even after downing a few handfuls of chips, the vigorous thumping in my chest continued. Then, my breaths came increasingly harder. I felt faint and had to sit down. I feared heart attack. Couldn't be. Too young. Just tired. Resting might help, I thought. I always think resting might help. But I rest as if it's a duty, a function to complete in order to "help." My mind doesn't rest. That day especially it kept up a fight. Painting must happen. Turnout must look good. *I* must look good. My child must be good. None of what was happening matched these criteria to my satisfaction. I was at war, all the combatants were inside my skull, and my whole body was on alert.

I assumed my physical discomfort would go away soon, a nuisance to be brushed off like a fly. It didn't. I casually told my husband, who had been spending more time visiting than painting, of my heart and lung distress. An ambulance? No, definitely no. I'll be all right, I told him; let's wait awhile and see what happens. Well, after we're done here, I can drive you to the emergency room. Yes, after we're done, after we've got more painting done. I sat and rested, some. I waited. I started playing with the children, to calm them down. They made me laugh. Then I sent them home with a friend and felt relief. I chatted with volunteers as they left and thanked them.

When the doors were locked, there was finally time to go

to the emergency room. I felt fine then. Calm heartbeat, easy breathing. Didn't seem necessary to go to the doctor, but . . . just in case. I felt foolish in the car on the way. My husband and a friend and I talked and laughed about the day. At the hospital, the tests said my heart was fine. I went home and slept.

It was months before this happened again—this strange experience of the fast-thumping heart, hard breathing, faint feeling, and all the rest, and more months of countless repeated episodes, some lasting hours and even days, before my doctor gave it a name and offered me medication. That gave me complete relief for a year or so, but not much longer. Therapy and all the other routes of recovery over the years have eased things and almost ended them, but not quite.

Panic attacks can happen anywhere, anytime. Sometimes an obvious stressor provokes it, often the cause is elusive. I've had panic attacks in my kitchen while cooking, in my bed when I've almost asleep, in meetings with clients, while playing tennis, in the middle of giving a speech, while hiking in the mountains. In most cases, I continue with whatever I'm doing at the time, as best I can. I can't always. Usually I have to drop out of a tennis match. Sometimes I need the herb valerian to fall asleep. I use other remedies that sometimes help. Seldom does anyone around me know what is happening to me. I don't tell others unless I think it will help me; it's too disturbing to entertain their questions and deal with their distress over the matter. Usually there is little they can do to help. Mostly I continue on, though in a more restricted way, until I can find a way out. Two episodes are most memorable.

The first happened one day when I drove 200 miles to give a workshop on how to gain peace of mind. It was one of a series of workshops I was giving all over the state for family caregivers. This one, sponsored by about a dozen health and social service organizations in a rural Minnesota county, had been promoted throughout a wide area. Dozens of people were expected.

I woke up that morning, the third day of a severe flu,

wondering if I should go, but clear that I must. I had no way to notify all these people that I couldn't be there. They were depending on me. It was the first day I didn't have a fever, so I thought I could pull it off. Realizing I was still weak, I asked a friend if she would drive me there and back, so I could rest on the way. I was glad when she said yes. I slept all the way there. Once we arrived, my friend dropped me off at the workshop site and left to explore the town.

When I went inside, I discovered that nothing had been set up in the room where I was presenting. No one was around to register people or to help me get the microphone and flipchart I needed. People began pouring in. I wanted to move quickly to get what I needed, but I could only move slowly, as a low fever flared. I managed to set things up, sign in registrants, distribute handouts, and generally prepare. I tried to visit pleasantly with people until everyone was seated. Thrilled by the turnout, I was also overwhelmed by the number of bodies in the room when my own body craved a soft blanket and tea.

It was time. The group quieted. I had to do this now. I gathered up my public presentation voice and manner and began the welcoming comments. Having polished this presentation well with experience, I was on automatic. I knew it was only three hours until I could go home.

Just as I got myself and the group hooked and motivated to go with me on this three-hour exploration, the back door of the room opened. In walked a woman with a television camera and notepad. A local reporter, she wanted an interview with me—now. Could I answer a few questions?

Not now. What was the matter with her? How could she walk in and expect this? Not when I'm trying to get a workshop in high gear. These people haven't agreed to this. I'm not prepared for this. Yes, it's true I want publicity for my work and my books, but not here, not now!

She persisted. We need it for the noon newscast, she explained firmly, expectantly, doing her job. At the end of the workshop, I said. I'll talk then. Before noon, she insisted. She wouldn't leave. My feverish brain stumbled to respond without losing my cool in front of this crowd who had gathered to learn about finding peace of mind. Agreeing to a prenoon interview would mean cutting the workshop short, I realized, and we had already started late. Squeezed, my resistance taxed to empty, I agreed anyway.

As the reporter exited the room, I realized I had been taking long pauses when trying to answer her demands, waiting for enough oxygen. At the same time, I was aware that a noticeable heart thump had been picking up speed in my chest. I worried it would be broadcast through my microphone. Stunned by the mix of fever and the lightheadedness from the attack that had suddenly slammed into me, I leaned on a table to steady myself. *I must go on.* I was hot and then chilled, losing my thoughts, hearing a zinging noise in my head. *Don't fall apart in front of all these people. Their lives have trouble enough. The last thing they need is to have come all this way and made all the arrangements to get here and then have to "care" about another sick person. Go on.*

I glanced to the side of the room where my purse were, where my pills were. *How can I get to them? The writing exercise is next. Just hang on until then. They won't be looking at me while they're writing. Okay, now go. Just get to the pills and pop them.* I feel like a junkie.

I knew the pills wouldn't work all that fast, but they gave me hope. I carried on through the rest of the workshop, teaching participants a simple process for achieving peace of mind in the midst of caregiving—the same twelve-step process used by Alcoholics Anonymous and Al-Anon. Recognize you feel powerless. Turn your life over to a higher power. Do an inventory of thoughts and feelings that interfere with your peace of mind, turn to your higher power for help in making amends for your failings and finding forgiveness, and maintain an ongoing relationship with your higher power and others who suffer and seek peace as you do.

The meditation I led them through toward the end, with the waterfall piano music in the background, soothed their spirits. It soothed mine, too, but only a little. I was too far gone. I prayed for help. My heart thumping sounded and felt like an off-balance load in a clothes washer. My head reeled off and on. I wanted it all to stop, I wanted to go home. I looked at the clock. *I must find the energy to finish. In time for the interview. Before noon.*

As people applauded, offered their thanks, bought auto-graphed copies of my book, asked questions, I sank beyond exhaustion. I smiled, said thanks, muttered practiced responses. As I bent over to sign books and then returned to full stature, each movement upped the ante with my heartbeat and my zinging brain. I wanted to pack up, to head home, and then . . . the camera. The interview. *I forgot!* I vaguely heard: "Stand here. Wait. Just a minute. Look at the little light. Okay, we're going live. What are some of the difficulties caregivers face?"

Caregivers? Difficulties? I was almost certain I would faint. I knew somewhere I had a storehouse of responses. I scrambled to connect the dots—fast. Stress, exhaustion, confusion, I said. Powerlessness, I said. Resentment, I said. "What message of hope did you offer them today? What can they do?" Higher power. Someone or something they believe in. Inventory. Notice what keeps them from peace of mind. Surrender. Blood rushed into my face and left as fast. I could tell another question was coming from the reporter's lips. I waited a long time for it to reach me. "Is there anything else you'd like to say to caregivers who may be watching?" Pause, pause, checking. No.

The light went out. The thumping in my chest was all I heard as I stood alone in the room, packing up. My friend arrived to take me home, and I could not speak.

I still sometimes have attacks that are this severe, occasionally right in the middle of an important presentation or conversation. After all the ways I've learned to overcome them, I feel like a failure at times for not being done with them altogether. Yet, I am also able to celebrate that they are less frequent and that often I can head them off or shorten them substantially. Perhaps most important, they don't frighten me anymore. Having survived that workshop experience and another experience during which the change in an airplane's cabin air pressure during a panic attack caused me to black out, I trust I will survive again. I have more experiences and resources to draw upon now.

One of the more helpful resources for me has been a book co-authored by Judith Bemis and psychologist Amr Barrada, called *Embracing the Fear: Learning to Manage Anxiety & Panic Attacks.* This book helped me recognize that, rather than trying to hurry up and get rid of anxiety when I felt it, it was more effective to stop and *allow* the anxiety to be there. The authors help identify the exact self-talk that goes on in anxious moments, and then suggest other self-talk that is more realistic; instead of "This is terrible. I *have* to stop feeling anxious," it's more helpful to say, "I am feeling anxious, and I do not have to change that." It's not all that simple to pull off when something threatening (real or imagined) feels imminent, but when I do follow this process, most of the time it works. It's a revision of the "hurry up" script that has plagued me since childhood and that often gets me into panic reaction in the first place.

In another memorable panic episode, I had a great opportunity to practice their suggestions. I was a few miles up a mountain hiking trail with a friend when panic hit fiercely with the usual symptoms: racing heart, difficulty breathing, alternating heat and chills, extreme lightheadedness, difficulty focusing, and anxious thoughts. Here I was, a long way from any kind of outside help, sizzling under a ninety-degree sun, and barely able to walk more than a few yards without collapsing. Walking, especially up stairs or uphill, exacerbates the symptoms markedly. In the worst attacks, the breath nearly gives out every few steps.

After a few minutes of "trying" to stop being anxious, I remembered what Bemis and Barrada had said. I began to notice my self-talk. Sure enough, I was thinking, "This is terrible. I'll never get down from here. I have to hurry up and get over this because it's late in the day and I have to get back to where we're staying before dark." There were several more "This is terribles," including, "This is spoiling my plans for getting to the beautiful falls today, and it's ruining my companion's hike."

As soon as I noticed these "terribles," I began to shift my internal conversation as gently as I could. "Yes, it's true, I am anxious, and I will probably be anxious for a while. Then I'll be done being anxious. If I can only walk a few feet at a time, then I'll walk a few feet and stop before going on. If we don't get to the falls today, it's okay. Nothing terrible will happen because of that. For now I'm feeling anxious, so I'll just allow the anxiety to happen."

Almost immediately, I felt the "pressure" lifting. I didn't have to hurry up and stop feeling anxious, I could just "be" with it.

I kept up the new mind-talk for a time, and then decided to experiment to see what would happen if I started walking onward toward the falls, albeit much more slowly. I was willing to turn around and head back to our lodge if need be, so I eliminated any "have to" that might create more pressure.

I walked *very* slowly at first, continuing to accept my anxious feelings, and not trying to rush any faster than I could comfortably go. Fortunately, my friend was supportive, readily adapting her pace as needed to accompany me. She was willing to go back down the trail to try to get help if necessary—though neither of us could quite imagine how I might be carted out of this tree-packed terrain if I had to be rescued. I concentrated on noticing what was happening, and just letting it happen. The more accepting I became, the less anxious I felt. Before long, I was at the falls, anxiety-free!

It felt like a miracle. Accept and go free. The exact opposite of every impulse I feel to escape fast, somehow, anyhow, when anxiety strikes. Accept it, don't fight it, don't create expectations that it will get better. Just stay with what is happening, and have *that*. That's what I did on the mountainside and I was almost giddy on the walk down. This was one of the first times I had ever been able to get through an attack without an outside intervention such as medicine, herbs, a homeopathic remedy, or some extended meditation or body awareness work. And, as if nature wanted to add its own reward, a momma bear and her babies strolled casually across our path, delighting us by their presence. Though I realized that danger was a possibility if we startled the mother in any way, I didn't even feel anxious! I had found acceptance.

I still use this strategy quite often. But sometimes I can't seem to get to that level of acceptance on my own. My thoughts are so anxious and scattered, and I become so discouraged and ashamed, that things feel hopeless. I struggle to find acceptance and it eludes me.

Once, a rash of panic attacks kept me on edge for much of a week. None of the usual remedies seemed to help. Acceptance was only a word. I did have a sense of trust that this terrible feeling would pass eventually, as it had always done before. But I felt alone with my distress, and *wanted* to be alone with it for the most part. When the intensification of the attack interfered with my walk with Brian, I told him that I wanted to go home and be by myself. I did that and felt better, but not much. Panic means I don't feel safe. Somehow my whole sense of survival feels under attack. It's a primal terror seeking a primal response, a childlike feeling of wanting rescue, wanting to be held.

That evening I was with two friends, Mike and Deni. We three had been meeting weekly for more than a year. (Later, the meetings continued with just Mike and me.) We had a way of creating a safe and sacred container for holding and dissolving one another's pains and limitations and for expanding our possibilities. A cup of tea and their company quickly sent me into tears. I was feeling in such despair after days in the war zone.

"I've been holding on, and I'm tired of holding on. I have this sense of wanting to let go, sink, melt, drop down like an elevator, stop holding on like I'm responsible for everything."

I crawled into the space between Mike and Deni on the couch. My head was cradled in Deni's large arms and lap, my thighs tucked close to my chest, and my feet draped over Mike's legs. Mike turned out the big lamp near us. I closed my eyes, and asked my friends to sing a soothing song to me. Both chose the same one by grace. "You are my sunshine, my only sunshine," they sang, as they gently stroked my arms and head.

It was dark. Curled fetally, I settled into the warmth of the womb. Mother and father, they took turns saying words of comfort to me while I cried and shook and sank down through my hurt for more than an hour. "You don't have to hold on. You can let go now. We'll hold you. It's safe." I must have felt safe when I was in my mother's womb, I thought to myself. I longed to remember, to return to that ultimate safety. I was crying because I'd forgotten how to float, drift, only breathe. But soon I was sinking, melting, dropping through, not responsible. The tears and shaking diminished. I was still holding on, but not as tight. I felt deeply loved, like I'd gone home, and a lot safer than before. The panic had left me.

I just wanted to feel safe. We all want that. For some of us, that safety can be suddenly snatched away. Just a wary thought wakes up old fears, old stories. Compassion, tenderness, waiting are needed; acceptance, surrender.

Chapter Ten

Say It with Eggs

*E*ggs come in very handy when you're angry. I learned that in my late forties around the time of my divorce. An acquaintance told me that she'd found the act of hurling a dozen or two at a tree to be therapeutic. It's not very demanding on the body (unlike pounding madly on a pillow or punching bag), no serious damage is done (unlike throwing plates at evildoers), and there's no need to dispose of the mess afterward either; the birds will handle that.

When the divorce was final, I invited my women's group to join me for an egg-hurling ritual to honor this mighty shift in my life. The group, begun in the 1970s heyday of feminism, had been meeting monthly for over a decade, attempting to claim what Gloria Steinem and Betty Friedan had declared was ours. We weren't bra-burners or men-haters, but the "Father Knows Best" families we had come from had crippled our sense of worth as women, and we were looking to take our rightful place. None of the members (except me) had abandoned long-term marriages, but most had gone beyond household duties to take on careers—teacher, lawyer, child-care center director, legal secretary. In our group, we had been learning together how to raise our own self-esteem, how to assume equal power in our marriages, and how to raise children of both sexes equally. We had taken care of each other's kids and been a refuge for one another when marriages weren't going well. We shared stories of assertiveness practice and therapy sessions. We even served as pallbearers for one of our members—an unusual role for women then. Our lives had been intimately linked.

With the help of these friends—along with countless books, courses, and lectures on codependence and equality—I had been able to grow myself a career as a writer, go back to complete my college degree, and even stand up for myself in my marriage now and then. Still, I was a long way from being self-assured— or many times even knowing what I felt or what I wanted. If my husband or a friend asked me what restaurant I wanted to go to, I didn't know how to figure that out. I waited to hear what the other person would suggest. I wanted to please—especially my husband, so he'd be happy. If he was happy, then he'd be easier to live with and—I kept hoping—he'd lighten up on our son.

How Ben treated our son was at the heart of our marital troubles. When it came to raising André, I had no trouble figuring out what I wanted. I believed deeply that children should be treated with kindness and respect, and I wanted to talk about that with Ben. I wanted to work closely with him to raise a happy, healthy, and confident child. But he wasn't interested in talking things over. He had his own methods for child rearing, ones that mostly I found to be harsh and intolerable.

Ben was a crowd-pleasing humor man in public, but often distant and sullen at home. He had little patience with our son. I would watch in anguish as Ben forced food into his two-year-old's mouth as part of his clean-the-plate insistence. I tensed up each time he threatened to "take your head off" if André spoke during mealtimes and interrupted Ben's almost perpetual TV watching. At dinner, I often drank muffled tears with my milk and swallowed my meatloaf and my hope through a constricted throat. As André reached his early teens, I remember gasping in horror one day (but silently so as not to be heard) when I saw this normally bright-spirited boy curled up in a fetal position on the couch, wearing the same look of fierce fury I had seen too many times on the face of his father.

I tried over and over to convince Ben that encouragement, rather than intimidation, is the best way to help a child learn, and that a small child can't tell ahead of time how much food he might be hungry enough to eat. I reasoned. I pleaded. I complained and explained. I offered him child-rearing books to read. I tried to hug or compliment him or guilt him into agreement with me. I always did these things "nicely," trying mightily not to make him angry. I was terrified of anger—his or anyone's. In my efforts to convince him, I was critical and manipulative and, I'm sure, annoying. I wanted him to be a kind and attentive father, and he wasn't buying it—not my version of how he should do it anyway. As the years went by, my fear mounted over what level his rage might reach if André ever became the slightest bit rebellious as a teenager.

By the third time we went to couples therapy, I had begun to despair. The therapy experiences would diminish Ben's ferocity to a simmer for a time, but before long his corrosive scowl, his hostile dismissal of requests to talk things over, and his tirades toward André would soon resume, making our household feel like an airtight chamber where the next breath might use up the last of the supply.

One night I called Sharon, my oldest friend and a member of the women's group, to moan about Ben's behavior. "I can't stand the way Ben is ignoring André these days. He walks right by him like André's a piece of furniture. The only time he talks to André is to yell at him if he happens to be in Ben's way. This has been going on for three months! It's driving me crazy."

Sharon, in her Scandinavian matter-of-fact way, had given me advice dozens of times before. She was a child-care center director. She knew a lot about kids. "Why don't you dish up the food for André and just give him a little at a time until he's full?"

she'd say. Or, "Take André to the other room at mealtime and eat there with him. Leave Ben with his TV." Sometimes I had tried her solutions. Sometimes I was too scared to.

This time Sharon's solution seemed extreme. "Don't tell me what's bothering you. Tell *him*." She wasn't scolding, just saying the obvious—the one thing I didn't want to hear. I drew a deep and rapid breath. If my familiar strategies of trying to win him over with niceness or reason didn't work, I thought I had no other choice but to cower or to complain to my friends. Now, Sharon was suggesting that I actually bring the complaint directly to him—straightforward, without the "niceness" and with no need to please. But meeting Ben's anger head-on felt to me like throwing myself in front of a train. My whole body tightened and I began shaking.

I couldn't bring myself to do it while we were married, at least not until near the end, and then only halfheartedly. I couldn't quite sacrifice the appeasing persona that I so fiercely thought I had to maintain in order to be loved. I continued to stay in the marriage for a long time because there were many things I admired and appreciated about Ben, and I believed it was possible we could find a way to be a happy family—if I just tried hard enough.

It took more than twenty-one years of marriage before I filed for divorce. I asked Ben one day, with my usual cautiousness, "Could you take André to his after-school activities more often this week? I've got an especially busy schedule these days and I've been taking him most of the time lately." In response, I met a blast of rage I could no longer stomach. It was the gift of my PMS at that moment that ruptured old restraints, flushing the outrage that had been surging through me longer than I could bear. Blood met blood. "That's it. I've had it," I announced. I left and went to see a lawyer.

But even through the divorce I stayed excessively civil and didn't ask for child support.

A few months later I invited the women from my group to join me for the egg ritual. That night I was still inhaling the fresh whiff of freedom—feeling light, confident, self-satisfied. Glad I had escaped, I took pleasure in being able to do so without getting nasty. I hadn't let this angry man turn me into a vengeful person. I had remained kind, pleasing. There *was* anger burning beneath the crust, but as usual I had carefully covered it in ice in order to keep cool and look good. But I didn't understand that then. What I did recognize was that I *had* felt some anger during my marriage, and I wanted a forum for airing those past grievances—a closing ceremony of sorts. Throwing eggs sounded safe, even fun. If some real emotions flew in the process, all the better—I felt entitled to cry out in righteous anger after all those years.

Sharon, Heidi, and three others arrived at my home that midsummer Friday evening, each toting a contribution for our dinner. They also brought two cartons of eggs apiece as I had requested, one for me and one for their own exclamations of discontent. Each of their marriages had rocky elements. After refrigerating their potluck offerings, we gathered up our egg cartons and took to the streets. We were headed for a small, creekside woods about six blocks from my house—a relatively secluded spot just right for this venting.

Though righteous emotional release was the intent for our outing, oddly silliness prevailed as we marched down the center of neighborhood streets in our jeans and sweatshirts. We seemed like restless teens trying out some group mischief for the first time. At times we strode boldly and spoke loudly, off to show the world that some dues were going to be collected that night. At other times, we pulled off an innocent casualness, even as our eyes occasionally cast about to spot possible onlookers who might find us out. After all, we were carrying eggs—hidden in grocery bags. Preparing for an act of vandalism. A little stealthy, a little edgy, a little excited. Is anyone watching? Can we get away with this? Our daring yet secretive mode was more show than real risk—we walked along mostly empty tree-lined streets with wide lawns and no one in sight. Yet, because this was the first marriage of the group to end—breaking the rules of our (mostly) Catholic upbringing—the occasion merited at least this small staging of adventure. Before long we abandoned caution and erupted into a full-volume, reckless chorus of "Oh-oh freedom" and "Gonna wash that man right out of my hair." I wished I had a good singing voice. I wanted my voice to be heard above the group, belting out my fury and freedom with a loud, clear, confident tone that would draw people to their windows.

By the time we reached the woods, it was near dusk. The small elm cluster we entered offered a suitable dark cover. We began to unpack our white missiles.

As we stood around and looked at each other, we became giggly and awkward. Here we were, middle-aged career women slinking into a stand of beautiful trees to hurl dozens of eggs. Were we really going to do this? Fortunately, Heidi, a short, talkative woman who was always ready for a laugh, pulled out of her bag several spray cans of colored stringy material. A few quick spurts created orange and yellow strands dangling and looping among the tree branches. We shrieked with laughter. Now we were officially vandals. A perfect warm-up for egg flinging.

I found just the right tree and planted my feet firmly. I drew my arm back, aimed, and heaved the first oval toward the tree. It missed and plopped soundlessly in cushioning brush. Not exactly the smack I'd anticipated. Laughter all around. All right, a little more gusto then.

Adding voice to gesture, I threw again, this time doing more of a baseball windup and taking more careful aim. "Here's to never having to please anyone anymore," I said in a test-run tone. *Wham.* A near miss, confirmed by dabs of dripping yolk on the tree trunk. Whoops and cheers cracked the air, spurring me on.

"No more living with craziness!" I said, trying to muster up a serious tone. *Wham.* Globs of yellow and white landed right in the center of the trunk. Applause and more cheers.

I gripped the next egg more firmly and reached farther back, wanting to grab hold of the fury I had held back in so many moments with Ben. "Enough is enough!" *Smack. Crack.*

Now we're getting there. For a moment I felt it, the belly pressure expelled, my vertebrae snapping into alignment.

I raised my voice.

"If you won't help me, then just get out! Get out! I'm through with you."

The windup was bigger on this one and the hurl more forceful. Still, my voice was barely at half-volume. I wasn't used to standing up for myself—certainly not loudly. And the silliness of the outing seemed to override the serious. But the words were spoken in front of witnesses, and my whole body had gotten into the act. I didn't have to be contained and careful here, denying or holding back the force of the fury I felt, and I didn't want to. Yet I was doing just that. All I could manage was a novice's clumsiness—letting a little of the tightness and terror I felt in cell and sinew have their say. In my Codependents Anonymous meeting, I had learned that when you want to practice new behavior, you have to start by "acting as if." This was my first rehearsal.

Yet, my missed tosses and timidly voiced feelings served as an invitation for others to join the frolic. They took up the hurling, some with even less precision and more hesitant voices than I. They weren't divorcing their spouses, but they had messages of their own to deliver. Sharon railed about her man's sullen nature, much like my ex-husband's. Heidi demanded more understanding from her husband. And the others made similar declarations, practicing, too.

We left the woods well after dark. Back at my house, we shared a wild rice chicken dish and fruit salad, then saged the house to purify it of its old stories. I remember feeling sated by the support of this caring circle of women that night. But after they left, I questioned myself: Had this all been just for show? After all, having staged this event to celebrate an emotional Fourth of July, I had only managed to light a few sparklers. And I had thought at least one tear would fall.

That was the first occasion I threw eggs. It was more symbolic than substantial—far from a heavy-duty cleansing of all my hurt. But I trusted the symbolism to deliver up substance in due time. And I was willing to keep practicing "as if." Whatever my limits and self-doubts on that occasion, what I remember most is my arm moving through space with force—and the smack of the egg against the tree trunk, putting the final exclamation point on the divorce decree.

Ten years later, egg throwing seemed like the right thing to do again, this time to help out a friend.

Nancy called me in a state of distress. She was experiencing some sizeable rumblings of anger. In the seven or eight years we'd been close friends, Nancy and I had both talked about how we had learned early in life to crush any semblance of anger. We had often bemoaned the fact that we hardly knew what anger even felt like. And now, during our midlife years, we were both exploring how to reclaim more fully this strange, uncomfortable emotion. That is, we had *talked* about the subject of anger and how important it was to recognize and deal with it in healthy ways. But when she called me that day, Nancy had clearly gone beyond talking about it; she was *feeling* it raw. Decades of outrage appeared ready to erupt, and I could tell she was both scared and excited. "I don't know what to do with it!" she said amidst her usual endearing laughter that thinly disguised panic. This bubble of anger was ready to burst.

I didn't know exactly what the anger was about; Nancy had never confided much of her troubled history, and she wasn't offering any details now. The cause of her anger didn't matter, but hearing her passion as she actually *felt* it made me excited for her, and a little envious.

"I know some people get rid of their anger by buying up a bunch of old dishes and smashing them," said Nancy, "but I can't imagine doing that. Too scary. Too messy. Too dangerous!"

Eggs. I remembered the eggs. "How about throwing eggs at a tree?" I told her of my earlier experience.

Nancy exploded with laughter. "Perfect!" she said. "Will you do it with me?"

"Yes," I replied immediately, glad to support her freedom and aware that I still had plenty of my own disturbances—old and recent—yet unvented. While I had made some progress in giving voice to my feelings in the prior ten years, my crushed self-worth was still under reconstruction. I still tended to look to others to make decisions about places to go together. I had a hard time setting limits when someone was pushy or annoying. Instead, I'd stuff my irritation until I'd accumulated more than I could tolerate and then mail a "Dear John" letter. And though a decade had passed, I would still tense up whenever I thought about the way Ben had treated André.

I had only a vague sense of all this when I agreed to join Nancy on the egg-throwing expedition. Mostly, I was excited for Nancy.

At six o'clock the next evening, we met at my house, planning to go to the same woods that had sealed my divorce. Though I lived farther away now, the safety of this secluded spot was appealing.

When Nancy arrived, we headed to a tiny nearby corner store to buy eggs. Lots of eggs. We wondered if they'd have enough in stock. They had plenty. But once it was time to actually make the purchase, Nancy hesitated. Her tall, big-shouldered body slumped. "I don't know if I can really do this," she whispered while flashing her wide eyes and a questioning grin my way.

"I'm just going to start with two dozen," she declared and

headed to the checkout. I decided to get one. She wanted to test this out small, and I thought twelve smacks would be adequate for my own irritations—at least for starters. I was still expecting the main workout to be hers.

Coming out of the store, we both glanced at a stand of woods next door to it, about two city blocks in size. I'd driven and walked by these trees many times, but hadn't thought of this place for our egg tossing. Yet there it was, offering a perfectly handy hiding place. Looking around first to make sure no one was watching, we walked past our cars and then, hunched over, we scooted into the woods.

The trees were dense, with thin trunks and low-hanging branches and vines, but we squeezed our way through to a small opening in the middle. The density created a dark protective cover for our mission. Perfect!

This all seemed quite absurd, of course, even for me, who'd done it before. Throwing eggs at trees! I still wondered, what if someone saw us? But there we were, heading toward Nancy's freedom—and maybe rubbing off a little for me.

Like my first tosses years earlier, Nancy's were wimpy and missed the target widely. Her smile of surprise when she saw how far off-target she had thrown spilled over into laughter.

The targeted tree was obviously too thin. We went in search of a wider one and found a tree with two trees behind it as backup. With half a dozen eggs now used up, Nancy finally landed one where she intended. Wide open eyes and a giant grin showed how pleased she was. We both laughed. I suspect she could have gone on tossing the rest of her eggs in this giddy state, and I soon recognized it was up to me to take the lead on addressing our more serious purpose.

I decided I'd get busy tossing a few of my own eggs. I wanted to show Nancy how serious venting could be done. Sometimes we just need to hear or see someone else do what we long to do in order to find the courage to do it ourselves.

After a few moments of scanning my mind and body for something that could serve as kindling, the image of Ben force-feeding André and berating him mercilessly snapped my jaws into a clench. I was there again at the dining room table, frozen, muffling my horror. No more, I thought, and a fire came roaring up through my body.

"Stop it!" I yelled, heaving an egg toward the target tree.

"Stop it! I won't let you do that anymore!" This time I yelled even louder, and threw with more force. I was not laughing. I was saying what ten years earlier I had been too frightened to say. When I looked at Nancy, her laughter was now gone too.

She took a deep breath, closed her eyes, then opened them again. Standing firmly in her full height, she released an egg toward the tree, beginning to give voice to her anger. "Leave me alone," she cried.

Then another egg. "Leave me alone!" This time she was shouting.

Leave *him* alone, I thought to myself. Waves of heat rising from my belly fired up my arm again, and another egg flew from my hand. "You had *no right to do that! You were wrong!*"

Nancy continued with her own tirade, "Get away from me. You don't own me!" With each throw, her volume increased, her toss became stronger.

"*I* decide! *I* decide!" she screamed, egg after egg flying, smacking, cracking.

Yes, *I* decide, too, I thought. It's up to me to take charge of choosing and getting what it is I want—and of stopping what I don't want. It's up to *me*.

More eggs were soon needed, and within a few minutes we returned from the small store with another five dozen.

Nancy and I both were now even more ready to draw deeply from the wells of anger and sadness and restraint we had carried within us for too long. We were ready to *feel* all that had frightened us and to give it voice.

"You fucker!" Nancy let loose, her usual embarrassment grin showing for a moment, then giving way to the fury she wanted to claim. "You fucker!" she screamed with passion.

I was excited for Nancy. I didn't even need to know who were her objects of rage, nor the stories behind it. I was simply ecstatic as I heard her chains falling away. I could feel and hear my own dropping as well. The nerves in my body vibrated with sweet liberation. For neither of us was this about a desire to attack someone else. It was rather the "no" we had not been allowed to say in our childhood families, and then had not allowed ourselves to say in other relationships. It was also the "yes" we longed to say to our own heart, our own strength, our own worth.

As the last of the eggs made their mark, we had moved from fury to exhilaration and celebration. We threw our arms up in the air and began dancing unrestrained among the trees. This was our day, this was our life. Our spirits soared. The rageful tones soon shifted into song. We created spontaneous lyrics and melodies that ranged from operatic to Broadway musical.

"Don't you," Nancy sang, pointing her finger playfully but decidedly at all those who would stomp on her spirit.

"Don't you," I chimed in, and then together we continued, "don't you, don't you tread on me. No, no, no [shaking our fingers at them], don't you tread on me." We sang as loud as we had yelled. We wanted the world to know that no one would trample us. We weren't going to allow it anymore.

At one point in our song making, Nancy interrupted, exclaiming, "You have a beautiful voice."

I said, "Yes, yes, this *is* a beautiful voice. I've never heard myself sound like this before." And it was beautiful. And I loved the feel of it rising raucously out of my throat. Here was a voice I'd never heard before—a full, clear tone, without edges or hesitation. While helping Nancy give voice to her rage, I had found a new voice of my own. It came forth, much as the chick breaks out of the egg, whole and vibrant, and here to stay.

A few weeks later, a woman berated me for not accepting and publishing a story she had written for a publication that I edited at the time. I heard myself trying very hard to appease her. Then heat rose from my belly and I told her again, but more firmly, "No." I didn't care if she liked me or not.

I drove by the site of our egg throwing a month or two later and was shocked to see that the entire two-block area had been cleared for a housing development. But in the midst of this stripped-down lot, three trees were left standing, right about where Nancy and I had let the eggs fly. Sometimes now, when I drive down that street, I glance over at those monuments to my liberation and break into song.

Part Three

Get Out There and Dance

⤝⤞

Creating movement is not effort, but fullness. Gestures draw us out into the room around us, allowing us to take up more space. We meet places where we hold and fold our bodies, and give them room to play. We tell stories, letting movement, sound, and stillness give witness to our loves and our longings. Unrestrained laughter and lightness of being are possible side effects of this experience. So is tenderizing of the heart.

Transcendental Bodies

*M*rs. Phebee was covered in black whenever I saw her, which was mostly at church. She wore a long black furry coat, a small black feathered hat, and black gloves. Even her rosary and her prayer book were black. She must have spoken sometimes, but I don't remember her uttering a word when she rode with my mom and me to church on occasion. I can't say if she ever smiled.

At church I'd glance over my shoulder and see her in the back pew where she sat by herself, learning forward to rest her arms on the pew in front of her and touching her knees to the edge of the kneeler. Unlike the rest of the congregation, she didn't stand, sit, and kneel with the rhythms of Holy Mass. Nor did I see her lips move during rosary prayers or Mass hymns. She was a static, dark, humped-over form.

But as Sister led the congregation in saying the rosary before Mass, I could see that Mrs. Phebee gripped her rosary tightly, shifting her thumb and forefinger firmly from one bead to the next. That was how Mrs. Phebee prayed, this simple gripping and shifting.

Prayer is often thought of as leaving behind the body to go into the realm of soul or spirit. That's how I learned about it anyway. In my Catholic upbringing, I was taught to deny my body in favor of my soul. The soul, the nuns said, was where God would be found. Yet the divine is often known and shown through the body. The sensory speaks *of* the sacred and *to* the sacred. In fact, despite the traditional denial of the body, some childhood church rituals are quite physical.

I, too, fingered my rosary beads over and over, not only at church, but nightly in the family living room where my mother insisted we all kneel and recite the Hail Marys and Our Fathers and Glory Be's. I had been taught in Catholic school that each decade of the rosary—ten beads side by side between single larger beads—represented one of the sacred mysteries of Jesus' life to be contemplated: Gabriel's announcement to Mary that she was to give birth to Jesus, the Nativity, the scourging of Jesus after he was condemned to die, the crowning with thorns. There were fifteen "mysteries" altogether. Each time I said the rosary, I worked hard to imagine and *feel* each experience along with Jesus and those around him. I tried to feel his sadness and fear in the garden the night before his death as he prayed to avoid the torture that was to come. I even tried to cry along with him. I imagined the sharpness of the pain as nails were pounded into his hands—wincing as if the nails were going into my hands. I stirred up surprise and joy as I imagined standing beside his friends as they saw Jesus again after finding his tomb empty. It was my way, in my own living room, to go beyond the sermons and the religion classes and the *Lives of the Saints* to *experience* a walk with God in the same way that Jesus did. Being on my knees, gripping my rosary like Mrs. Phebee, and reciting the ancient, repeated prayers with feeling were the disciplines of the body that gave entrance to redemption.

In church, I practiced kneeling, genuflecting, and silence as signs of reverence and readiness for more of this Godly experience. On Christmas Eve before Midnight Mass, the dark stillness in the church, broken by the choir's "Silent Night" and the candlelight processional, raised goosebumps on my arm and sent a wash of sweetness through my body. I was there at the stable, welcoming my Lord.

Every time I attended Mass in childhood—daily except Saturdays—I looked forward to Communion. As I received the tiny tasteless wafer on my tongue, drew it into my mouth, and let it dissolve (we weren't allowed to chew it), it became one with me. I believed as I was taught, that this was the body of Christ—not in a symbolic way, but the real thing. Not that the bread was supposed to take on the physical characteristics of Christ's body—that change was in the mysterious realm, the realm where God could do things, through a priest in this case, that humans on their own could not. When taking the Christ wafer into my mouth, I liked having the chance to be in touch with Jesus in this physical way. I felt like I was inviting him in and bringing him close to my heart. There was silence afterward, a time of getting to know him better now that we were joined in this special way.

At other times of the day, outside of Mass, I would just sit in church in the presence of God, as if I were meeting him at a park bench and we were friends, getting together to have a good talk. I knew God was there because the Blessed Sacrament—the leftover consecrated wafers from Mass—was kept in a chalice inside the tabernacle right at the center of the main altar. This gilded tabernacle was God's home, and the Blessed Sacrament was evidence he was there. I genuflected and stayed silent out of reverence.

I almost always attended the day of "adoration" on the first Friday of each month. The Blessed Sacrament would be "exposed" in a shiny monstrance, a gold stand with pointed projections of varied lengths emanating from the center, much like a brilliant star. A wafer, no longer hidden inside the tabernacle, was visible through a small circular window at the star's center. On the day of adoration, God, in this form, was not to be left alone; people signed up to sit in the presence of the monstrance for hour-long periods. An hour of sitting was a long time for a child, but the sparkly monstrance and the thought of being responsible for keeping God company lured me to sign up. And there was the promise of indulgences—a chance to lessen the time I would have to wait to enter into heaven after death if I died with unforgiven sins.

As I sat there in the big silence of the massive church building, the sights and sounds around me helped lead me into prayer. The shiny monstrance, stained glass windows, stations of the cross, and statues of Jesus, Mary, and Joseph fostered my devotion to God. Rows of red candles in front of the statues especially attracted my eyes. They were white vigil lights actually, appearing red in their crimson glass holders. The flickering flames and shadows were the only things moving during the hour I was there, except for the occasional turning of prayer book pages. If I had a nickel, I'd put it in the slot on the side of the cast-iron candle stand and light another candle. I loved to watch the flames reaching to pointed peaks and then shifting shape again and again. Beyond their physical beauty, the candles provided a hands-on form of prayer. By lighting them, I paid homage to Jesus and the saints, and sought their favors.

Every religion has its rituals that bring the sacred into the domain of the flesh. Buddhists assume meditation postures, become students of the breath, and practice mindfulness in daily activities. Native American rituals incorporate rocks, branches, and other objects from nature. In one ceremony, the sun dance, metal hooks are dug into a person's flesh. Muslims prostrate themselves in prayer five times a day facing Mecca. These are the outward expressions; their physicality is a way to bring heaven to earth. Some religious expressions, such as the use of fire and music, are so universal that they seem elemental to humanity's spiritual experience.

Belief in, or a longing for, some other dimension of existence beyond the tangible is clearly more than a mental exercise, a thought-out decision. It's built into our cells. Some scholars have recently claimed that a sense of the spiritual is merely a brain and chemistry response—endorphin arousal, like a runner's high, prompted by certain physical activities or by stimulation of the imagination or by an emotional attraction to love and companionship. We "feel good" and we embue this feel-good quality with a transcendental meaning. But perhaps this inborn cellular impetus actually confirms that our every neuron is directed like a compass toward a compelling, magnetic, numinous force.

It's said that walking a labyrinth, a religious practice for many centuries, draws the participant into a profound experience of the sacred. Despite my usual attraction to things sacred, I must admit I was skeptical when I first heard about the labyrinth. How could simply walking in and out of a maze-like configuration offer anything more than good exercise and maybe a headache? As I looked over a huge labyrinth design painted on a retreat center parking lot one day while on a retreat, the narrow pathways struck me as confining. I thought I might get bored walking this repetitive pattern, or I might take the wrong path, like in a maze, and get frustrated. Still, toward the end of the retreat, I decided to give the labyrinth a try. Obviously it must have some merit, I thought, since so many people I respected found value in it. And if my walk wasn't going well, I could always quit.

I had been advised to go into the labyrinth with an intention, a prayer, or some problem to solve. I mixed all three. Since I had a vexing problem on my mind, my intention and my prayer were to solve it. I had volunteered to be a group discussion leader during the retreat, and the group I led was delightful—except for Reverend Nagia. A black Ugandan minister, Reverend Nagia was the only clergy member in the group. I prided myself on an appreciation for diversity, but I had a problem with this woman. She had a formula for everything.

Though she was pleasant enough and clearly sincere, she annoyed me when she "preached" to the rest of us about what "one must" do. In my judgment, she wasn't there to learn and grow like the rest of us, but to proclaim.

As the days went by, she continued to rankle my peace of mind. It wasn't only her declarative approach that bothered me; I found my own intolerance of her upsetting. After all, maybe this was a cultural difference I should learn to appreciate. From what she was saying, she seemed to be a respected elder in her community, one sought for guidance. Perhaps she was just doing what was right and natural in her role back home. However, I didn't think it was her role in this situation, and I clearly wanted her to change. I wanted her to comply with the group guidelines, which were to speak self-reflectively rather than as teacher or preacher for one another. I had tried gingerly to encourage the prescribed approach, but she either didn't understand me or wasn't willing to conform. As the week progressed, I felt anything but the love this retreat was designed to foster—at least for Reverend Nagia. I hoped the labyrinth walk would give me words I could use to help her see things rightly—loving words, of course.

I noticed that several people were already walking the labyrinth, at different speeds, causing the need to pass each other in the narrow pathways. I felt nervous about that. If I were to enter into a spiritually transcendent state, I didn't want to bump into people and have my ecstasy disturbed. Nevertheless, though unsure and unsteady, I took the first step. I walked slowly—it seemed the spiritual thing to do—but not too slowly. My usual rush to completion was tugging at me.

As I had expected, the walking seemed boring and confining at first. My mind wanted something to do and soon got lost in its own internal maze. *Should I be going slower? Faster? How many turns are there in this thing? How is that stiff little woman over there going to benefit if she rushes through it like that? Am I lost already? This is going* to take forever. I kept walking. *Why isn't Reverend Nagia out here doing this? Maybe she'd lose some of her righteous attitude. There must be something I could say that would let her know she's out of line, without hurting her. I wish I were better at this group-leading business when people aren't cooperating. She's missing out on the discovery and mutual support that come when people are vulnerable and share their honest self-reflections. I should be able to help her do that, as the leader.* I kept walking. *This is taking way too long; all that's happening is that I'm getting more upset with her.* It seemed like I'd been walking an hour or more when I reached the center of the labyrinth. There I should stay for a while, I had been told. There something would happen.

As I lifted my foot to step into the center, I saw out of the corner of my eye Reverend Nagia. No longer a misplaced pawn in my mind, she was there in the flesh, just a few feet away, walking as I had been walking. She seemed smaller than my mind's image of her, unassuming, and flowing in her movements. This woman who had disturbed my sense of safety and security because she hadn't been following the rules the way I wanted her to, who had seemed inaccessible, even defiant, was now walking out in the open, searching, like me.

I stood in the labyrinth center and waited to see how God might touch me. It happened quickly. I felt the demands for her compliance slide off me like a heavy belt dropping away from my waist. My flurried thoughts stilled and, for the first time, I felt care for her arise in my heart. My eyes softened. My jaws loosened. I gazed at her with compassion. *She is just acting in ways that help her feel safe. She is fearful and fragile, like me.* At that moment, I wanted to hold her and tell her everything would be all right. The love I was feeling didn't demand change.

My heart has long been on a quest to open wider and steep itself in this kind of love—the kind I think God is made of. Others assure me I'm a loving soul, and I've spent much of life in helping others. Yet there is a difference between simply doing things for others and doing them with feeling. It's like giving money to save a forest but never experiencing the smell of pine. Love is a physical experience, and without the physical, it tastes like saltless bread. I want to feel the love, to have it swell my heart to overflowing. Too often, though, my heart feels closed down. At times, I have sunk into considerable self-reproach and even despair over my lack of warmth and caring. And as I've gotten older, I'm even more aware when my giving feels like going through the motions instead of an act of the heart. I don't know why my tender feelings are so sparse. Maybe being brought up with too many rules, or with more shame than acceptance, has limited my ability to feel caring emotions. Maybe I suffered such disillusionment and grief after my marriage failed that I shut down my heart in self-protection. What I know is that when my heart is "full," when I feel love and appreciation wholeheartedly, it is usually because something of the divine is shining through.

On a later retreat at this same center, I found myself bemoaning the closed feeling of my heart, aware of the many ways I shut myself off from others and hesitate to give. I wondered if I'd ever catch on. Though I made an appointment to see a spiritual counselor to discuss my distraught feelings, I wasn't very hopeful. I had tried many times to discover how to soften my heart, with limited success.

"Come in," said a gray-haired, middle-aged man in a boring brown suit. "My name is Jerry. Please sit down." In his small, poorly lit office, he looked like every out-of-date minister's portrait I had ever seen hanging in church corridors. "How can I help you today, Pat?"

I didn't know how to answer. *Tell me how to love. What's wrong with me? Why don't I feel God's love within me?* How could this man, in one hour, answer such questions?

"I don't know how to love," I said. "If I were really close to God, I'd feel God's love. I'd be able to love the same way that God loves. But I feel dead inside."

"What do you mean, dead?"

"I go through the motions. I try to be loving. I pray. I meditate. I try to be close to God. But I don't feel much in the way of care for anybody, and it all seems phony. I don't even feel connected to God very much, even though I want to."

Jerry gave some prescribed answers. *Just let God love you. Maybe you're being hard on yourself. Do you think love is always a "feeling"?*

This was going nowhere. I was sorry I had come. Jerry was talking, but I only feigned listening. I just looked at him. I could tell he was sincere, but fumbling.

"What do you think would help you?" he finally asked when it was obvious his offerings were a misfit.

I waited for an answer to come.

"I wonder what Jesus' heart would feel like," I heard coming out of my mouth. I was taken quite by surprise. I rarely gave much thought to Jesus at that time in my life. My religious beliefs had changed since childhood, and while I still considered Jesus to be a wonderful spiritual teacher, I was much more interested in the ways God showed up in my everyday life than I was in this historical person. So his name seemed especially odd to hear and the question about his heart even odder. I looked around as if somebody else had spoken it.

Suddenly, I felt something pushing out from inside my chest—a huge thickening, as if a large lump was growing and pressing up from under my ribs. It felt too big for my chest cavity—the size of a small cantaloupe. Warm, pulsing, it was moving like a baby inside a belly. And it felt full of love—more love than I could have ever imagined. I sat there, silent, tears flowing.

"I can feel it. Jesus' heart. I can feel it inside of me," I said finally.

Jerry didn't say much. He just sat with me while I let in the love.

Because my heart knew the experience of that moment—an experience that stretched out over three or four days—I am able to remember. It is there again, as I write this, the large heart in the chest cavity of my body. It is the physical and the transcendent together.

～

For us to know transcendence, it must take physical form in some way. Artists—visual and performing—perhaps understand this better than most. Their creations often express a spiritual experience. Nancy Chinn, a watercolor artist interviewed by Robert Wuthnow in his book *Creativity and Spirituality*, describes how her work is guided by a spiritual impulse that literally *moves* her: "I just start out with a gesture, almost like a yearning, a prayer. I don't plan these paintings ahead of time. They're a way for me to see what my intuitive side looks like with me working as the witness to what happens with the paint." Her comments remind me of a vine compelled to sprout blossoms and bear fruit. The beauty emerges because it must.

The transcendence does not belong to the artist alone; its physical expression can spark in viewers or audiences a set of responses mixing the sacred and sensory. "When I dance," says liturgical dance artist Jamel Gaines in Wuthnow's book, "I'm abandoning myself [to the point that] I can touch someone in the audience. It will make a difference, and they'll be like, 'That was just breathtaking—not even just because you did five turns, but just the way you reached out and the subtlety and the beauty of that and the spirit of the face and your chest and the way your legs move, I just feel like *I* could have gotten up there. You represented me up there.' That's who I do my art for." Who among us has not been elevated into divine communion from watching such a dance performance, peering at an exquisite painting, or hearing music that rang through us?

That same access to transcendence is available within each of us, whether we are artists or are engaged in house painting, loan processing, or child rearing. A pervasive divine energy lifts us beyond this world even as we are immersed in it. What that calls for is the "abandoning" of self that Gaines mentions—a submission to the sacred force streaming through us.

Buddhists speak of mindfulness, bringing full, detached attention to our every experience. From this perspective, every act, every physical engagement—from washing dishes to listening to the phone ring—holds the promise of a revelation and an enjoyment of the numinous. Even without action, simple awareness and appreciation of the physical world, our own body included, can become an encounter with the sublime. The respected Buddhist teacher Thich Nhat Hanh, in *Touching Peace: Practicing the Art of Mindful Living*, speaks of consciously noticing our eyes, blessing them and marveling at the miracle of sight. He talks of attentively appreciating and caring for each of our body's organs: "Our eyes are us. Our heart is us. Our liver is us. If we cannot love our own heart and our own liver, how can we love another person?" One of the early New Thought teachers, Myrtle Fillmore, describes in her writing how she cured herself of tuberculosis by spending extended periods of time each day blessing specific parts of her body and thanking them for their wonderful work. Loving attention to our physical form changes it, and changes how we live. As Hanh says, "We do not have to die to enter the Kingdom of Heaven. In fact we have to be fully alive. When we breathe in and out and hug a beautiful tree, we are in Heaven. When we take one conscious breath, aware of our eyes, our heart, our liver, and our non-toothache, we are transported to Paradise right away."

When, in the art class I took in my twenties, I was asked to spend ten minutes lying face down in the grass, with eyes open, it was one of the most "eye-opening" events in my life. I met with studied gaze (mindfulness) what I had walked over for years with little awareness: the sculpted forms and bends of the grass blades, the varied hues of living and decaying, the smell of green juices and soil, the wide assortment of tiny, busy bugs. My response to this paradise was reverence, ecstasy. I had gained entrance into the Kingdom of Heaven. I painted with ease and joy for the rest of the class.

Historically, at least in some religious traditions, the separation of body and soul has been emphasized, but the body may be the primary doorway to, and for, the divine. In fact, what *can* we know of the transcendent without our bodies—at least in this lifetime?

ᕲ Chapter Twelve

Hangin' Out

I suffered for many years from neck tension. Meditation, relaxation, massage, Feldenkrais lessons, and many other therapies had helped intermittently, but the tension reappeared every morning. It showed up as I drifted out of sleep and typically camped out most of the day from the base of my head down into my shoulders. The price I had paid over the years was enormous. Not only did I experience persistent pain and discomfort, but the muscle constriction often crimped my ability to play tennis or paint a wall or even carry groceries. My many attempts to find a way to "relax" my neck had also cost me thousands of hours and dollars.

A few years ago, I decided to attend an all-day Essential Motion workshop led by Karen Roeper. I signed up mostly because of my thirst for the fun and freedom of creative movement, but I was aware that Karen had even more to offer. A longtime dancer, dance teacher, and student of the body, Karen had developed a reputation for helping people uncover and dissolve emotional blocks through heightened body awareness. By midday, I was feeling relaxed, playful, and refreshed. After lunch, Karen offered to do one-on-one somatic coaching. When she asked for volunteers, I decided to find out if she could help me free the tension in my neck. I raised my hand and walked up to stand beside her as the other thirty participants looked on. I was nervous yet excited.

Karen's calm, clear manner had gained my trust during the first half of the day. She had led us through a series of improvisational movement activities that provided a comfortable warm-up for the afternoon coaching. The first hour of the morning we stretched the ways that dancers do, gently coaxing every major muscle group, and some minor ones, into greater agility. Then, gradually, Karen prompted us to begin moving about the room, however we felt like moving, oblivious to others around us. There was no need to perform or please anyone but ourselves. At first I hesitated, stymied by intermittent flashbacks of a teen-age ankle sprain from doing the Twist and being asked to dance at school parties only by guys performing an act of charity. Yet Karen's gently reassuring instructions slowly slipped in past my memories of clumsiness. Soon, dreamy music prompted me to drift into a silvery state of consciousness, with no agenda but to let my body lead me. Little by little, I eased into exploring the pleasures of leaning, dipping, lunging, curling up, rolling, and resting. Other bodies moved around me in a mirage-like blur, and sometimes another person's way of leaping or bending or twirling piqued my interest. But mostly my attention was on my own body. I would watch and feel my one hand rising or my one knee bending, as if in slow motion. It felt like being two years old again, discovering what happens when you move this way or that.

At times, Karen played spicier music and guided us in moving bigger and faster, sometimes alone, sometimes joining our movements with those of others. I found myself in a spirited communion of dancing, weaving webs, shadowing the lifts and leaps of others, and then being followed and mirrored myself. The overall experience of the morning session was mesmerizing and exhilarating. I felt agile, free-flowing, energized.

The one-on-one coaching session began after lunch. After telling Karen briefly about my neck tension, she suggested I go ahead and feel the tension there fully. Intrigued, I complied. I

stopped my usual effort to relax the muscles and simply observed the feeling in my neck. My shoulders rose and drew inward. My jaws tightened and my teeth clenched. I was startled
and self-conscious about what was happening, but I was also
curious. Karen reassured me: "Just stay with it. Trust your body."

I decided to close my eyes, paying closer attention and
avoiding the distraction of thirty pairs of riveted eyes. The
tightness moved down my torso, front and back. It kept inten-
sifying. This seemed so odd. I wondered if this strange tension
would take over and not leave me.

"Just stay with it. You're doing great, Pat."

I felt my chin dropping and my cheeks spreading wide into
a grimace. The muscles in my forehead and around my eyes
tightened. My body seemed ghoulishly disfigured, like a Dr.
Jekyll or Dracula. What was happening felt out of my control,
yet I also knew that I could reverse it if I wanted to. For now, I
was drawn in, as if falling through a hole into Wonderland, and
I offered no resistance

From my solar plexus upward, everything became tighter
and more contorted. Tension descended into my arms, which
rose behind me, the palms of my hand facing backward. The
movement was so intense and extreme that I felt as if someone
else had taken over my body parts, moving me like a muscled
marionette, but from the inside, rather than with strings.

"Stay with it. Follow where it's going."

My shoulders pushed up toward my ears and my head dropped
back toward my spine. My arms pressed harder backward, as if
against a wall, while my upper torso pressed forward in opposi-
tion, yet the impetus for this intensity arose from within me. I
was a pressure cooker, with insides pushing mightily against—
nothing.

In this contorted state, I tried to explain to Karen what was
happening, "It feels like I'm pushing, very hard. It's very uncomfortable. It hurts!" I was straining as if my life depended on it. I

hated this feeling yet felt at home with it. It was some terrible yet unnamed truth I had been living, that my body had been crying out about for a long time. My eyes were wet.

"What are you pushing?" she asked. Her question was so obvious, simple.

"Nothing," I answered. A vast stillness followed. Almost at once, the accumulated pressure began to dissipate.

I stood there, quietly stunned, taking in fully the absurdity of what I'd been experiencing—pushing when there was nothing to be pushed. It was so familiar, this making of my life a struggle, everything taking enormous effort. I had lived that way for years—for all the years my neck had been complaining. Shopping for a new car when exhausted, on a below-zero day, rather than waiting for better conditions. Driving long hours on trips without stopping—having to "push on." Trying endlessly to make a marriage work that just wouldn't.

"Maybe there is nothing to push," she responded quietly, echoing my words but amplifying their meaning. My whole musculature had already begun to register this very notion. The painful pushing sensations rapidly subsided. Tension dropped away. I felt myself standing taller. I was not pushing.

For a moment, I stood there, still, surprised. In a few minutes that seemed timeless, I had allowed myself to fully experience a range of feelings that my body had been aching to reveal for a very long time. The tension that had nagged at me had had its full say, forcefully enough that I got the message, and it was no longer needed.

I opened my eyes and looked at Karen's smiling face. I told her about my tendency to push my way through life. At her suggestion, I said a few times, "There is nothing to push." With each repetition, that notion sunk in further. I felt lighter. I smiled bigger. Relief. Big relief. I was almost laughing.

"Now walk around and experience what 'nothing to push' feels like," she suggested. I tried to comply, but when I lifted my right leg to take a step, I felt off balance. I couldn't figure out how to move my leg or where it was going to land. This was a new body I was working with, one I hadn't experienced before in motion, one that wasn't tight and pushing. Everyone in the room could see how I was fumbling, and we all laughed together as I wobbled my way through new steps.

To my surprise, the biggest shift in my body was in my pelvic area. Everything below my waist was noodle-like. I began walking, but it was not walking as I had known it before. It was more like gliding, my whole body *easing* across the room. "I'm feeling like I'm just 'hangin' out,'" I said with a broad smile. "I've got hips!" I thought of young street-corner dudes with nowhere to go, whose whole bodies sway widely side to side as they move on down the street. No pushing, just *hangin' out*.

At this point, I was giddy. The whole group was laughing with me amidst breathy sounds of surprise.

After a while, I sat down, and it became the group's turn to mirror back to me what they had seen. They all stood and I watched as they tightened and contorted their arms and torsos the way I had done. Their faces showed mounting anguish as they took on the imprisoning tensions. Watching this multiplied mirroring in front of me, I was deeply moved by the pain. Compassion permeated my whole body—compassion for myself, for them, for all who experience self-torture born of fear. It flowed from my heart—my large heart—out of control. As I watched their fumbling attempts to walk newly as I had done, I smiled and cried and longed to help them the way I'd want to help an infant making her first steps. In these emotion-laden moments, I knew I could forgive a lifetime of missteps—my own and those of others.

They accumulate—these trips and falls—as we make attempts to get what we long for. Our psyches and our bodies bear the bruises. If we're hurt often and badly enough, they wisely conspire to protect us from further injury. They form and position themselves to avoid such dangers. It's a matter of survival.

My mother pushed. Not in a mean way mostly, but in her daily, insistent "hurry up and do what you're told right now" manner. With nine children to feed and bathe and keep out of danger (after losing two in infancy and having another nearly burned to death), she pushed to create order, compliance, safety, and security. I learned from her to push, too. *Life is hard. You have to work hard. You have to push to get what you need. An idle mind is a devil's workshop. Hurry up. Get moving . . . or else.*

After driving myself for decades by dutifully perfecting the skill of pushing, my body became weary and registered its protest. It could no longer bear the tension of this distorted intention, and it asked for mercy.

As I witnessed the group reflection of my experience, I felt drawn to redeem the innocent—myself and all humankind. What have we all done but try to make our way in the face of fearful autocrats who live around and within us? Even at age fifty or sixty or ninety, we're only trying to learn how to walk with ease through our world, to pick ourselves up if we fall down, and not to get hurt again. Compounding that are the years of distortions that our bodies cry out for us to notice. We try to be strong, look strong, and bear ourselves as nobly as we can. But we have bent shoulders, carved into submission from too much shame, or jaws tight and aching from—perhaps—anger unvoiced and unresolved. These and other signs of body anguish tell of a fragility often attributed to aging but more likely the result of living out misjudgments about our very nature.

I saw such de-formations in the family of bodies before me. While they acted out *my* pain, some of their *own* wounded ways of moving and holding themselves showed through. They no doubt had encountered errant rulings by their own parents and other punitive forces, and convinced themselves of what they must do to survive, to get along, to succeed.

Such wounds can fester for a long time before they emerge as pain, sickness, or disease serious enough to require a doctor's visit and perhaps lead to a life sentence of misery. This gathering provided an occasion to attend to them well before they got that bad. Kindhearted attention allowed us to reset our bodies so they could move with ease again.

When the mirroring process was finished and the group sat around me again, I felt a pervasive tenderness for each person. They had all accompanied me into my secret places. They had shown me that they understood. Every face smiled back at mine. For the next few minutes, we talked about what had happened. I remember most a comment from a man named Tom: "This morning you seemed like an interesting person to have an intellectual conversation with. Now you seem warmer, more approachable." I imagine that's because I had stopped pushing. I was just hangin' out.

My experience in this workshop reminded me of Scamp, a dog that André had when he was young. Scamp was picked up by the city pound once when he left our yard. After he returned home, it was clear that something awful had happened to him while he was away. Scamp curled up in the corner of the yard and recoiled whenever I offered him food or called him to come play. Somebody had evidently treated him harshly, and now he couldn't trust even those who had always treated him well. It took almost a week of frequent, gentle reassurances and gradually moving closer to him each day before his frolicky, fun spirit was revived and we could all romp with him again. It was a lesson in not pushing. Nothing could hurry his recovery from fear. Nurturing attention and reassurances of his innocence and safety restored his trust, but that happened only because this process was applied over a week.

After Karen's workshop, I had hoped that my newfound feelings of looseness and freedom would become permanent. But as with Scamp, time and repetition have been necessary for this sense of ease to take hold. I haven't been able to rush it or push it, not after decades of well-trained self-constraint and contortion. But since that day with Karen, I have become more attentive to how my body feels as I go through my day. I try to be alert to what's tight, what's loose, and what wants to move, letting my body instruct me. And each Friday noon I gather with a small community of friends in a yoga studio for a weekly ritual of improvisation dancing. We give our bodies permission to move freely, to dance, to play. We savor the chance to let our bodies have their say.

Fear is possessive, settling deeply into the body. But it can yield in the presence of attentive, accepting kindness. Noticing—without judgment—where the body's movement or resistance seems to be, is a holy act. Within an ongoing practice of reverent attention, whether through meditative and creative movement or other mindful means, the body responds, encouraged to romp, or just hang out, until these pleasures become natural and body and spirit feel at home together.

๑ Chapter Thirteen

Born to Be Wild

> Our bodies are wild. The involuntary quick turn
> of the head at a shout, the vertigo at looking off a
> precipice, the heart-in-the-throat in the moment
> of danger, the catch of the breath, the quiet mo-
> ments relaxing, staring, reflecting—all universal
> responses of this mammal body.
>
> —Gary Snyder, *The Practice of the Wild*

*N*ewborns are wild. Arms and legs flail. Screams erupt. A
baby's whole body responds instantly to a tender touch
or sudden prick. Watching a newborn, I warm to this wildness.
I am drawn to its newness, untamed, vibrant. Surely my own infant wildness was once as engaging. My parents and my broth-
ers and sisters must have tickled the bottoms of my feet just to
see my legs and arms flail in response. They must have delighted
in my spontaneous squeals as they cooed to me. As I grew, they
must have thought it "cute" when my wildness became more intentional and I tried to grab for something shiny and fell down.
They must have encouraged me to try again despite the risk.
Later, these same people civilized me, insisting that I sit still and
be quiet and behave. They contained my wildness so it would
not disrupt their lives and so I could fit in and get what they

thought I needed. I was carefully taught to control my nature, and even to forget it.

Gary Snyder, in his book *The Practice of the Wild*, rewrites each definition of "wild" found in the *Oxford English Dictionary*, breathing a newborn vibrancy into them. Among his remakes of the word's meaning are:

"Of plants—self-propagating, self-maintaining, flourishing in accord with innate qualities."

"Of behavior—fiercely resisting any oppression, confinement, or exploitation."

"Of behavior—artless, free, spontaneous, unconditioned. Expressive, physical, openly sexual, ecstatic."

My Christmas cactus fits those definitions. It branches freely and randomly, well beyond the edges of the pot. It vigorously defies gravity, pushing upward, flourishing according to its inward impulses, and "fiercely resisting" any confinement. It is expressive, physical, ecstatic, and even openly sexual as it flowers.

Still, it requires water, sunlight, and the nutrients of the soil, which it pursues with persistence, stretching its branches upwards and sinking its roots. The wildness of my cactus is not lived in isolation, but amidst a web of wilderness where energy is exchanged and allegiance to nature's ways is required. No moisture, no nourishment, no sunlight, and the cactus will die.

It is dangerous being wild. The *given* must be *given up* in order to get beyond it, and the price is unpredictable. That risk is part of the attraction, sometimes a compelling attraction. It is also what frightens me and makes me want to play it safe. But when I resist the surging wildness within me, the danger I seek eventually finds me anyway.

In my early forties, I signed up for an intensive six-day personal empowerment program. The program included a ropes course. This involved being strapped into a hanging device attached to ropes and leaping off a cliff across a cavernous opening, trusting the ropes and the support of fellow participants to assure a safe landing. Even though the course was designed to be "safe" if everything went according to plan, plenty could go wrong if the demands of nature weren't meticulously respected. The possibility of injury or death, though highly unlikely, gave the experience an edge. I would be pressed to face the core fears that were holding me back from living my dreams. The leap off the cliff would require surrender of body, trust in teammates, and a willingness to transcend assumed limits.

Thrill and terror rushed through me when I signed up. Could I at last break free from the confinement of hypercarefulness that had overprotected me since childhood? Could I feel the freedom of flying through the air, abandoning all need to hold in and hold on? Could I survive, let alone endure, an unnatural drop into space? And once I made the leap, how would it feel when the straps holding me yanked my back and shoulders sharply as gravity made its rapid and sudden tug? Having had years of treatment for back and shoulder tension, I tensed up fiercely at the thought of such jarring. Massive self-preservation set in. *I cannot do this.* Then I learned that those with a doctor's "excuse" would be allowed to skip mounting the ropes. Their role would be on the sidelines, to encourage and assist the others who were taking part. That, I decided, I could manage.

Relieved, I immediately made the required appointment for a pre-course physical with a medical doctor. While my chiropractor, who had treated me many times for back and shoulder pain, might well have endorsed a restriction on swinging from the ropes, the allopathic doctor saw no evidence of a problem on my medical clinic charts. I pleaded and convinced him to take X-rays despite his seeing no clinical reason to do so. The results reiterated his opinion: the few muscle spasms I had now and then would not put me at any special risk if I did the ropes course.

But I was desperate. Beyond the genuine concern for potential injury, I felt a far more gripping terror of losing control—of being dropped and falling into my wildness. As much as I longed to fly, my eyes told the doctor, *I cannot do this.* No, he *had* to give me that excuse. And I convinced him. He signed the necessary form. I would not have to step off the cliff.

⌐

When it came time for the ropes course, I was assigned to a support station a few hundred feet below the jump site. Two others joined me. We didn't have to jump. Our job instead was to yell words of encouragement as the jumpers swung out across the cavern and down past where we stood. As assistants for the course, we too were expected to put our "life" on the line, by giving all we had in the way of spirited support. We were not to hold back. We were reminded that those facing the terror of the ropes and leaping into the wild were counting on us to believe in them.

Waiting for the jumps to begin, I was half wishing the doctor had stood firm. True, I would now have been facing the greatest terror of my life—loss of control—but this would also have been my chance to break through it. Unable to remake my choice now, I decided I could at least grab for a leap in spirit. Abandoning my midwestern reserve and be-quiet upbringing, I surrendered to the assignment the course leaders had given us—to provide unbridled, enthusiastic cheering for those making the jump. I went "wild." I started to scream, "You can do it! You can do it! Go! Go!" I clapped and whooped as the first, then the second jumper sailed by. As though cheering someone on for the Olympic gold, I jumped up and down, throwing my arms high. Suddenly, overcome with an exuberance that craved a reach beyond gravity, I leapt with my slim body onto the back of the broad-shouldered man in front of me. Though surprised, he nonetheless stood firm, but I wasn't able to establish a grip. I slipped off and landed on my tailbone. I was in great pain. It took weeks for my body to heal, and even longer for my psyche.

Wildness is risky. I longed for the freedom of a leap through space, yet I avoided the ropes to play it safe. I conserved my wildness while craving its full expression. This tension plunged me into another kind of danger zone. Leaping in my own way, I did so explosively and in isolation; I didn't have supports in place as the jumpers did. I let myself go, but didn't notice where I was going. I expected more of myself and the man in front of me than nature allowed at that moment. The knowing of my own nature had been frayed since childhood and I got a blunt new lesson as I hit the ground. Wildness and recklessness are not the same thing.

At age fifty-six, I joined the circus for a day. I signed up for a two-hour Introduction to the Circus class after watching a theatre performance featuring stunning, sensual women climbing, tumbling, lunging, swaying, and flying in exquisite, free-flowing dance among low-hanging ropes, long, draped cloths, and trapeze swings. These were women flush with grace and grittiness who also kindled a sense of hearth-like ease and subtle mystery, women I could trust. More than a dozen years beyond my escape attempt from the ropes course requirements, I was sure I was ready for adventure now. If these women could do it, so could I. At least I could attempt Circus 101.

I was excited when I showed up for the class. After years of chiropractic treatments and massage, physical therapy, body awareness activities, strengthening exercises, and tennis playing, I felt looser and more agile than I had ever been. Even as I looked around at the other students, many of whom were gymnasts and dancers, preteen to midtwenties, I was not deterred. The trapeze dancers themselves were probably pushing forty. If they could do it, I told myself once again, so could I.

I had been a clumsy child—overweight, awkward, last one picked for any sports team. I couldn't skate, hit a ball, or shoot a basket. Always, I longed for the feeling of gliding through space with ease, my arms and legs flowing in smooth movements. I craved the cheers and backslapping after a home run or a perfect drop through the hoop. I wanted to belong. But more and more, I had shied away from even trying. I wasn't willing to fail again and endure the pitying and rejecting glares of my playmates. Instead, I went from awkward child to rigid adolescent. A "bad" back stiffened me well into adulthood. Yet, freer-moving now in my midfifties, I was loose enough for lunging and leaping, I was sure. At last, I would be able to feel the full freedom of flying that I had only sampled when pumping myself high on playground swings.

This was no small dream. In my office where I write, facing me every time I look above my computer screen, is a piece of ribbon hanging on the wall. On this ribbon is a treasured image, hand-sewn by a friend, of a girl in red flying upward with head, arms, and feet thrown back, her hands gripping a trapeze swing. That's me up there. My body has been asking to do this since I hung from tree branches as a kid. It is not out of reach. Sam Keen, in *Learning to Fly,* proved that to me when he took up trapeze flying at age sixty-one and made quite a success of it. Five years younger than him as I sat in this circus class, I thought to myself, *Why can't I?*

The circus women weren't there to entertain me. They were ready to make fliers out of me and the rest of the group—in one afternoon. After a swift round of stretches, we moved right into somersaults. The circus women demonstrated, exuding ease and confidence. Then it was our turn. Line up and go. This was definitely not a lecture class.

One by one, the tiny-waisted preteens and the limber dancers flew head over heels. I stepped forward to take my turn, bent over, and put my head to the mat. The rest of my body was supposed to follow over the top of it. It didn't. My torso twisted to one side, my head to the other. I felt a pinging sensation in my neck. Out of the circus teacher's bag came an ice pack, and I sat sidelined until it was time for the cartwheels.

I wasn't ready to quit, though. Buoyed by the seeming ease of the demonstrations and by the other students' willingness to be less than perfect in their attempts, I stepped forward and threw myself onto my hands. My legs never got more than a few inches off the floor before landing. No better than I'd done as a kid. Though my neck was still pinging, I decided to try again. The circus women supported my legs this time, but I had too little thrust and lost momentum halfway through. My body crumpled awkwardly onto the floor. I didn't care. I wasn't looking for anyone's cheers now. I wasn't even especially concerned about achieving a graceful performance. What I wanted was just to be brave enough to be in the "show." And maybe, just maybe, if I kept at it, I could experience a few moments of flying.

The exercises got harder and the directions swifter. We were asked to face a wall a few feet away from it, put our hands on the floor in front of us near the wall, and throw our bodies up in the air until they touched the wall and could lean against it. After a couple of attempts at this, I succeeded. There it was, that moment of flying, not knowing if I would make it, just letting my body go and feeling wild.

Ready for the big time, I took on the next challenge. A few feet from my partner, facing his back, I was to bend forward, plant my hands on the floor just behind him, then thrust my legs straight up in the air and continue on over my partner's shoulder and back, as he rounded himself forward and eased me along with him. I was to slide on and over his back and land on my feet on the other side of him. It had looked easy, fun, even magical when demonstrated. One of the circus women would be standing next to my partner, ready to assist me when my legs went up to make sure they were well positioned for arching over.

My partner looked tall and sturdy, confident. I was primed for the thrill. I had seen it work. I could do it. But the moment I placed my hands on the floor in front of me, I knew that something beyond the physical movements would be required of me. I hadn't quite been able to find that something in the somersault or the cartwheel. I had hesitated partway through on those attempts, cautious, wondering if I'd get it right. This time I knew there was no stopping place. I would go over and that was that. But first I had to thrust. Really thrust. Without holding back. I had to surrender to the movement and to trust that someone would be there to land against and someone would be there to steer my legs. There would be a moment when my body would feel out of control and I couldn't stop it. This was the thrill I had been waiting for—the freedom to thrust myself into the air with abandon and trust. I had always thought it was the flying that would be the thrill, but now I knew it was the moment of decision that offered the ultimate excitement—the leap to make the leap, the choice to take the risk, the willingness to give my body the freedom it had longed for.

As I readied myself for the launch into space, the circus guide asked me which of my legs I thought would come up first. She wanted to be prepared to catch and guide it. I didn't know my body that well. I'd never had this experience before. I took a moment to imagine how the move might go, checking for bodily sensations, and said, "The right one." "Okay," she said. Then it was time. I took a deep breath, and up I went, surrendering all. The thrill was there in that moment of surrender. I was willing to fly! I was on my way!

But it was my left leg that went up first, and my unpracticed thrust was a little short. Before the circus teacher could reach the leg, it dropped back to the ground and I landed on it awkwardly, twisting the ankle muscles severely.

The circus teacher was kind but didn't pamper. As she handed me the ice pack once again, her matter-of-factness sunk in: "This isn't easy stuff. We get hurt a lot, too."

This was the lesson I had missed on the ropes adventure.

Being wild is not only about the feeling of freedom. The risks are real. You get hurt. Willingness and surrender offer no assurance of protection. Even creatures at home in the wild have plenty of scars to show for it.

I sat out the building of the human pyramid that ended the day of circus initiation. I would have come back another day for more, if the circus troupe hadn't left town.

> There is a story of Coyote watching the yellow autumn cottonwood leaves float and eddy lightly down to the ground. It was so lovely to watch, he asked the cottonwood leaves if he might do it too. They warned him: "Coyote, you are too heavy and you have a body of bones and guts and muscle. We are light, we drift with the wind, but you would fall and be hurt." Coyote would hear none of it and insisted on climbing a cottonwood, edging far out onto a branch, and launching himself off. He fell and was killed. There's a caution here: do not be too hasty in setting out to "become one with." But, as we have heard, Coyote will roll over, reassemble his ribs, locate his paws, find a pebble with a dot of pitch on it to do for an eye, and trot off again.
>
> Gary Snyder, *The Practice of the Wild*

With age come increasing scars and deformities from cuts, injuries, habits, and illness—ranging from a surgical marking to the results of a fall to a decayed tooth. Some of these distortions result from accidents or deterioration over the years—life gone wild around and within us, out of our control. Others stem from moments of boldness—intentionally living wild. Each represents a wisdom story of damage, risk, and recovery.

During the Writing Your Own Permission Slip class that I teach, I guide participants through writing a "scarry" story. I ask them to close their eyes and pay attention to a particular scar on their body, recalling the story of how it came to be. Then I ask them to imagine palpating, caressing, and caring for it. I invite them to give their scar a voice and to have it write them a letter, in which the scar talks about all the wisdom it rep-resents—wisdom about pain and healing, injury and recovery, vulnerability and perseverance, risk and adventure, fracture and renewal, wounds and wholeness. Having done this exercise my-self now many times, I find each time I revisit and hear from one of my scars, it tells me something I could not have understood when I was younger. Somehow my scars get smarter with age.

When I first did the exercise, in my fifties, the "scar" that spoke a wise-with-years message was a collection of belly stretch marks from pregnancy. When I became pregnant at age thirty, I had spent the six years of my marriage building up the men-tal and emotional framework for remaining childless. I simply wasn't mother material. I had no interest in babies. Besides, I shared public concern about overpopulation. If I had any la-tent maternal instincts, they were quite well satisfied by tending to the hundreds of children in the neighborhood arts center I was running with Ben. My husband, having all the children he wanted from his first marriage, agreed with my decision.

When I learned of my pregnancy, I was horrified and ter-rified. I had to make a choice. Nothing in me would allow for abortion, though I gave it thought. Yet having a baby meant giving up the life I had planned (I couldn't imagine then how much my son would bless me). I traded the wildness of childless freedom to enter the even wilder unknown of parenthood.

When I did the scar exercise more than twenty years later, my life was on the verge of more uncontrollable changes. My stretch marks had a different message for me:

> I am the mother scar, the marks that let your womb make room for a son to rise within you. I came to teach you

about loving what you could not control and the lesson
is not over yet. You had to give yourself over to me once
and let me have my way. I stretched you beyond where
you wanted to go, beyond where you thought you could
go. You had no mothering in you, so you had to make
it up, create an opening for it, find the maternal mystery.
You are still being stretched, as your body and your
whole life change with age, and as your son now leaves
home. You can go into it, let it take you. It does not matter if your belly changes shape or you have more scars
to wear. Imagine what new son may be rising within you
that you cannot control. Imagine how it may bless you.

In attempting to shed the "be careful" lifestyle my mother
had taught me, I sometimes forget to take important precautions—exhibiting recklessness or even denial in the name of
freedom and wildness. That's how I ended up pregnant. That's
also how I acquired another unchosen scar a few years later. I
didn't check myself over for disease-inflicting deer ticks after
spending a weekend at a friend's cabin in northern Minnesota
woods. Within a few weeks, Lyme disease had me. I endured
high fever, profound and pervasive aching, and an agonizing
sense of depletion. *And what if the antibiotics don't work?* The attentive and loving care of my friends was my daily salvation.

Toward the end of this time, I again taught the class. This time
the still prominent rash scar gave me this message to write:

I came to visit you to teach you compassion. You have
been asking for a long time to be more loving, giving,
compassionate. Now that you've been in so much pain,
you know the pain of others more clearly. Your friends
with myelitis and fibromyalgia, chronic fatigue and
arthritis—suddenly, their pain is your pain. You know
their weakness, tiredness, difficulty moving, fears, and

tears. You hear them with new ears. Your heart is open.
You know how you felt cared for and how that saved
your life and softened your strain. You learned from
your caregivers the meaning of kindness. Once I leave
you, don't forget. Keep the love alive. It is what ulti-
mately will save your life and bring you home.

Living in the wild with full freedom means respecting how
nature works. Failure to know the body's strengths and inclina-
tions can lead to falls. Birth control neglect can lead to babies.
A lack of attention to real dangers can cause illness. Wildness
without wisdom can be fatal. Perhaps we can only acquire that
kind of wisdom if we dare to test our wildness and live long
enough to let it teach us. Newborns don't know how dangerous
their world is. Their impulses are wild. They reach for poison if
it glitters. They teeter along edges where they might fall. Over
time, they are tamed, in part so they won't get hurt. Yet, some
wounds are worth having. And living too safely contains its own
kind of risks. Falls happen and bones break from the brittleness
of disuse as much as from brazenness. Either way there's a risk of
shattering. But like Gary Snyder's coyote, we can pick ourselves
up and reassemble the parts.

Chapter Fourteen

Writing from the Body

*M*emory is a sensory experience. Something in the body percolates at the recollection of getting our first job or that "look" from Dad or Mom. The longer we live, the more memories our cells record. To write about the past requires access to it through the body. And with aging comes a compelling longing to tell one's story. As a person who sometimes teaches and coaches writers, I am often approached by people over sixty who say, "I want to write a book." What they mean is, *I want to tell my story, to leave my legacy. I want other people to learn from me. I especially want the people who mean the most to me to know that my life mattered, and to know what mattered to me.* That's why memoir-writing courses have waiting lists.

I think of Cookie Packer, a member of my Toastmasters Club. At eighty-three, she was losing health and memory, but not spirit. She never missed a meeting except when hospitalized, and she always came in laughing. A short woman with plentiful gray hair, she dressed in bold and brash outfits, always with a showy matching hat. Generous-sized jewelry dangled everywhere. Here was a woman who lived large in her small body. Her arms flew when she spoke. Her face displayed a thousand funny stories. Whenever she was scheduled as speaker, she brought props ranging from whistles to toilet tissue.

When Cookie wrote her personal story, it had to be a hands-on experience. She spoke of pulling out photos and drawings and certificates to prompt her memory. She fingered her collection of over one hundred hats, and brought out of closets her old jewelry, awards she had long ago received, and a collection of ceramic plates she had made. She showed us a selection of these items along with mocked-up pages from the book in progress. As she physically handled her "past," her stories re-emerged on paper.

Assembling the book itself was an ongoing physical experience. Cookie involved women from her church, who helped her spread her materials across church basement tables and arrange by hand each page to include not only typed copy but drawings, snapshots, newspaper clippings, letters, and other physical evidence of her vibrant life. During her last days, as she endured intense pain from the cancer that killed her at age eighty-four, she spoke with giddy anticipation about being wheeled to the local copy store to proof the nearly 200 pages that eventually were spiral bound into an inch-thick book. She died knowing her story would live. Indeed, it pulses through the pages.

I'd like to age like Cookie, with so much zest for life that my story would pulsate on paper. Thinking, by itself, doesn't do it. Core cell vibrations must ripple through a writer and shake themselves out onto the page. Writer's block may just be the jammed transmission of what the body knows. You just can't get to it because you've been sitting too long in a frozen position at the keyboard. Even when the writing is done by hand, being hunched over a table or seated among cushions in a near-fetal curl can stymie word flow. Something has to wake up the body's memory. Something has to *move*. I can't imagine Grace Paley writing her *New Yorker* piece called "Travelling" simply from factual recall. She must have felt her body refolding itself—at least slightly—as she described her memory of holding the baby of a weary fellow traveler:

He was deep in child-sleep. He stirred, but not enough
to bother himself or me. I liked holding him, aligning
him along my twenty-year-old young woman's shape. I
thought ahead to that holding, that breathing together
that would happen in my life if this war would ever end.
I was so comfortable under his nice weight.

In *Wild Ride,* Bia Lowe recalls, "After hours of playing in the
barn, the insides of my ears, eyes and nose were caked with
powder, and the back of my throat tasted of alfalfa." Surely she
had to feel dry and dusty while writing it.

If we are to write of memories, they have to reclaim posses-
sion of our bodies. That's why writers often go back to visit the
places they wish to write about. They want to smell, hear, see,
touch, and taste the milieu that contained the experience. These
sensory revisitations awaken the sleeping stories. Sometimes
all that's needed to tap these same body memories is mindful
attention. The job of the nonfiction writer, says Scott Russell
Sanders, is "bearing witness." What better place to start than
one's own body.

Unlike Cookie, for whom it came naturally, I need to remind
myself again and again to bring my whole body to my writing
place. It's not as if it isn't actually *there*, of course. But I'm not
always aware of it, *in it*. I once took a lesson in the Alexander
Technique (a posture guidance approach) in which I told the
teacher how tense my shoulder muscles get when I type. She
had me sit at a table, as I would at my computer desk. The first
thing she asked me to do was to *stop* and *be there*. She spoke of
end-gaining, the notion that we are always ahead of ourselves,
doing what we're doing with the next activity in mind. We also
tend to bring our last activity with us, replaying in our mind
what just happened or seeking solutions for a problem not quite
resolved. Our first task, if we're to be a witness, then, is to be

here, in the present, in our bodies. How can we bear witness to a past experience by writing about it unless we are first fully present now?

The next thing the Alexander teacher had me do was to be conscious of the whole space my body occupied and also the space I had available around me. It wasn't just my fingers and wrists that I was to bring to the job, it was my entire body. She reminded me to notice my breath moving throughout my whole body. She encouraged me to stay aware of my peripheral vision and my surroundings even as my attention turned to the computer screen. As I did these things, I somehow felt more of myself there, with more focus and yet more connection with the chair, the keyboard, the *space* around me. The energy available to tap the keyboard came not just from mind to hand but from my whole being. I was fine-tuned, every vibration in resonance. This state of body awareness and connection opened a clear channel to cellular memories. It is in such a state that I am able to "hear" again Cookie's loud laughter and allow it to lift my face into a smile. Then I can truly write about her *with feeling*. And more and more of my recollections about her can emerge on the page.

In my course, Writing Your Own Permission Slip, the body is honored as the teacher and vehicle for revealing the stories that compose our lives. Among various activities of play, movement, imagery, and drama, we play catch, not only in a circle but internally, in a game I call "belly ball," where we toss a ball of air back and forth inside our torsos. Something awakens when we do that. I've had the experience of finding spaces inside my body that I've been holding still since Dad or Sister Mary Rita told me to, years ago. And I've found remembrances of breathing large over triumphs and of sobbing deeply over losses I have known. There are treasure chests inside the skin, holding volumes dusty and sacred. Released from prohibition, they tell of secret dreams and agitation to fill plenty a memoir page.

Students in the course write their stories and reflections with a rapid ease and gripping authenticity as they bear witness to their body talk. After learning a few self-defense maneuvers to help them practice the art of saying no, for example, students describe a long-lost pulsing energy flowing through them and write essays in which they take an adamant stand for their lives. Past, present, and future stories all live in our bodies.

The antique hurry-up clock in my nervous system has a chance to get reset when I lead the class session on "time." Among the exercises is an experiment in walking observation. We walk at different speeds—the speed at which our life is going, the opposite speed, a variety of speeds, and finally the speed at which we'd like our life to be going. Usually, I am walking slower at the end, welcoming a reprieve from the deeply engraved impulses that are still too often carrying out the orders of the high-speed, demanding mother voice. This walking exercise is designed to help me and my students tune in to our bodies' natural rhythms. Yet, aware that I'm a novice at listening to my body and prone to excessive thinking, I don't fully trust my choice. Am I slowing down because I *should*? Am I truly noting my own somatic preference or choosing my new pace in defiance of the mother-voice? These present "stories" about myself and time, some of them fostered by past conditioning, are worthy of exploration and perhaps ripe for revision. Before I move myself—and the class—into writing our stories about the notions of time we live our lives by, I find it necessary to shift attention from head to heart.

The heart is not only a major rhythm center in the body, but according to scientists at the Institute of HeartMath in Boulder Creek, California, it also gives off an electromagnetic emanation that spreads out as far as ten feet away. It has intelligence and power, these researchers say. I say it does, too, not only from the Jesus-heart experience I had when I spoke to the spiritual counselor about my search for love, but because I've checked it out many other times. This power and intelligence go even beyond the physical.

I remember a few years ago working in an office with a woman who unnerved me. She stared into space a lot, her answers to questions were often evasive, confusing, and abrasive in tone, and she was extremely defensive. Knowing she had serious mental health problems, I tried to overcome my feeling of discomfort around her with compassion. Yet I invariably felt edgy every time I had to talk with her.

One day I sat down with her to talk about changes she'd need to make in order for a project to go more smoothly. I didn't think she'd understand or agree. In fact, I expected to hear one of her nose-in-the-air cutting remarks. I dreaded the thought of an ugly meeting.

Then I remembered an exercise I had learned from a course sponsored by the Institute of HeartMath. I decided to try it. I dropped my attention from my thoughts to my heart and felt my breath moving through that area. I continued the experiment by recalling a positive feeling (in this case, appreciation for a gift my son had given me). Already feeling calmer, I asked my heart how to be effective in this meeting and lower my high stress level. Almost immediately, I felt a flood of love for the woman. My heart had responded to my request by *softening me*. I was able to relax and speak with ease, clarity, and nonjudgment, and to my surprise, the woman responded in kind. It was the most satisfying conversation I ever had with her.

In the Permission Slip class, following the experiment in walking at various speeds, we do a writing exercise. The instructions are to complete the sentence, "When I let my heart set the tempo of my life . . ." Having come to trust the wisdom of my heart more and more, I am always eager to learn what it will reveal. Here is the unedited version of what I once wrote during this five-minute class exercise:

When I let the heart set the tempo of my life, there is a softening that surfaces, rising to the top, then wrapping like a comforter around me, cushioning me for a free fall. I am not keeping time. I am out of time, removed from the illusion of time as my executive director. I sink into myself, and on through the universe that is timeless and that will never let me fall too far. I am safe with my heart. I am on time with the pulsing of the planets and the slow rising of yeasted ground grain. And I am on time with shooting stars and the blinking of fireflies. No clock counts on me. I rise and fall on rhythms from within that rest or rocket me.

The heart carries a wealth of wisdom. So does our chin, our navel, our sciatic nerves. Staying awake to the nooks and nudges of our bodies can stimulate a healthy practice of writing as well as feed its content. Whenever I'm stuck with my writing, whether journaling on the couch or sitting in front of a computer screen, that blockage is usually accompanied by an urge to move. My body wants to be in on the process. Too often I read that internal nudge as a call to eat or drink, and respond by overfilling my body. But that is a disservice to me and the creative process. I'm better off if I get up and start dancing, or spend some time doing dishes or tending to my flowers. Even better, if I can, it helps to touch or do something related to what I'm writing about. If I'm writing about illness, picking up my thermometer or medicine bottle drops me back into the collapsed state of high fever and the despair I felt over the Lyme diagnosis, or reminds me of the beaches and winter warmth of Orlando because I once had to go to a strange pharmacy there to pick up some pills. If I'm writing about the canary I used to have, I open the laundry room cabinet where the aroma of a half-empty bird seed package perks my ears to half-hear again the warble that always grew louder whenever I talked on the phone.

Writing is a physical act. We are not done writing the whole truth until we're through breathing life into it, squeezing it into form, riding its rhythms, rocking it and letting it rock us, dripping with sweat. We have to taste and smell and touch the subject matter so completely that its sweetness and smoke and grit have hold of our hands and tap the keys. We cannot do this until our body opens its treasures and we are willing to take notice.

Chapter Fifteen

Bear the Body, Bare the Soul . . . And Let the Dancing Begin

Sometimes on all fours, sometimes upright, I would walk around as if I were a bear, feeling bulky—four or five times my normal size. My movements were large and lumbering. Occasionally, I lifted myself to full height and growled.

As I child, I often imitated animals that way, readily assuming their features. At age fifty-seven, I again took on the form and feel of an animal, this time a mammoth grizzly, a creature I had encountered a few times on mountain hiking trips. I had always admired, yet kept my distance from, the grizzlies when I spotted them among the pines. Frightened as everyone else by stories of maulings, I had come to appreciate the urgent closing of trails when one had been sighted.

A grizzly looks no more dangerous than a spaniel when I spy it eating huckleberries or romping with its young. Yet its huge size commands a cautious respect, and when stretched to full posture with paws ready to strike, the grizzly demolishes any childhood images of cuddly teddies. It takes up space, claims what it chooses, and noisily defies any other creature's interference. For a few minutes, while mimicking this huge mammal, I welcomed the chance to embody these same characteristics—to take up space, to claim what mattered to me, to let the world know my boldness.

The occasion for my bear imitation was a weeklong dance improvisation retreat. Offered by the Group Motion Dance Company of Philadelphia for members of the public, the midwinter retreat, which was held at a small dance studio in Sarasota, Florida, proved to be an irresistible invitation for me, warmth-deprived and movement-restricted as I was in the Minnesota cold. When I arrived at the retreat site, I met Manfred Fischbeck, the company's artistic director, and a dozen other people who also had come to Sarasota for this unusual dance experience—most of them, like me, well over fifty.

Having us mimic animals was one of many movement "structures" that Manfred used to guide our activities during the week. These structures allowed us to play and create freely within the many possibilities of movement. They gave us a chance to explore sensations, perspectives, and relationships in what he calls "the language of dance." Manfred and another musician improvised musical sounds to support and respond to our movements, using keyboards and a collection of percussion and wind instruments, ancient and new.

In the role of a bear, I felt as engaged as a curious child, eager to explore and experience how this animal feels, moves, and makes noise. Unlike a bear, I was raised to live small. The less space you take up, the less chance you'll offend someone. Cowering is safest. It means you're humble. Always defer, don't argue, especially if someone is bigger or louder or more insistent. Don't get anybody mad at you.

Moving across the dance floor like a bear, I tried on its largeness. Used to darting around quickly in a body slight of build, I was now spreading myself wide, feeling thick and heavy, and moving my huge limbs in massive, lumbering sweeps. Able to expand my sense of size and sway this freely, I felt in charge, invincible. No need to stay small now. As I assumed more and more of the hulky stance I had seen in the grizzly torso, my shoulders broadened and my clawed "paws" extended their grasp. The primal drumming, and loud, low, pressing keyboard tones pushed me deeper into the realm of nonhuman creatures. I bared my teeth. *Who dares stand in my way now? Who will try to shame me or hold me back? Let them beware!*

Years of niced-over hate and rage that couldn't find voice in a kept-small body at last had a stage. I did not even need to imagine the scoldings and rejections of my childhood, the resistances and hostilities in my marriage, or even the self-restraining "I can'ts" that so often kept me cramped while I craved to live life out loud. Rather, compressed cells throughout my body staged a rebellion. After a lifetime of moaning and groaning, my stifled cries found a new, untamed form—a series of growls as ferocious as my human voice could make them.

After a while (all sense of time was lost) of living a bear, I heard Manfred's words floating through the raucous music, "Now, shape your animal into a person." Slowly, I found myself taking on a burly male character—a pompous, back-slapping, cigar-smoking sort of fellow with a blustering *har-har* voice spouting off as if I were highly knowledgeable and in charge. Following Manfred's next direction, I wove among the other dancers, communicating as if I were this new character I had assumed. The others had also taken on humanized animal forms. We spoke to each other with the language of movement combined with mostly jibberish sounds, but in tones and rhythms befitting our characters. I took man-size steps, swung my arms out wide, formed my face into a fierce scowl, and growled out commands.

Like the week's other improvisational activities, this one led me to a subtle new awareness, not only of my body, but also of my psyche, spirit, and ways of relating. I encountered my grizzly, know-it-all arrogance, which I usually try to keep hidden, even from myself. This puffed-up bossiness showed itself in full force. It was harmless, of course. No one was intimidated by my show of dominance. No one was even watching or listening. The other dancers were absorbed in playing out their own animal-human representations with equal vigor. But for this little while, I embodied and enjoyed this overbearing posture, living it as big as I had tried to keep it secret. By giving expression to this shadow side of myself, I was able to get acquainted with it intimately, be playful with it, and shatter the shame I felt about it.

This show-off, bulldozer manner of mine has frightened and embarrassed me since childhood. I remember being told by adults and peers alike, "Don't be so bossy." I have seen people balk when I acted like the definitive authority on a subject or dictated directions rather than made requests. In my internal theatre, this survival-by-dominance stance is a natural opposite to my "humble" persona that lets others rule my life. Previously, I have tried to squash this overbearing approach. In this dance, it finally had its say. Now, it scares me far less than it used to.

I have come to love improvisational dance for the sheer joy of it. Movement emerges from what my body desires, not in pursuit of an outward goal or specific form. There is honesty, freedom, and authenticity in that. The body teaches us who we are. Even when a dance leader suggests a structure for the dance, such as taking on an animal character, that form becomes yet a further invitation for self-emergence. What animal will reveal itself? What does the body want to express?

Sometimes this type of dancing leads to the playing out of dramas like those revealed in the bear dance—the longings and endearments and shadows that linger within the body because they cannot easily be recognized or expressed in day-to-day life. Creative movement offers a playground for experiencing the lifelong, full-bodied exuberant study of life. I think Ashley Montagu in *Growing Young* was right when he said about people in their older years, "We should be encouraging the retention of growth of that freshness of spirit and outlook which the curious child, newly exploring the world with wonderment, delight-fully exhibits with what often seems like ecstasy."

At the Sarasota retreat, the animal imitation exercise took place well into the week. By then, after many rounds of stretching and dancing and playing in a variety of guided activities, I was feeling a remarkable sense of freedom and confidence within the palpable mutual trust of the group members. We had danced alone, in pairs, and in groups, bending, swirling, and intertwining in ways I had only tasted previously in a few other communal dance experiences. Once a very klutzy kid and still quite awkward on a typical dance floor, here I was swimming in delight over the exceptional fluidity, strength, and creativity of movement. Somehow, Group Motion Artistic Director Manfred Fischbeck was making dance—well, not *easy* for me, but *possible* and highly pleasurable!

A frequent and favorite activity during the retreat was a structure called "active-passive." One person "sculpted" a partner while the partner remained passive with eyes closed. What struck me about this experience was how tender human beings can be toward each other. What typically started with something as simple as lifting someone's hands or turning a person's head often evolved into a gentle stroking or carrying of this precious being.

Ed was often my partner during the week. This large, thick-necked, massively-shouldered man with a lumbering walk reminded me of the hulky bear I had been getting to know earlier. But Ed had no apparent growling tendencies. He was soft-spoken and wore a gentle-jowled smile. I always felt cared for in his presence.

In one active-passive exchange, when it was my turn to be passive, Ed lifted me like a child and placed me in a crosswise position on his lap. He placed my arms up around his neck, and rested my head on his chest. Like a father holding his little girl, he rocked me tenderly for a long time. Music coming our way took on a lullaby quality. Within this nurturing moment, all the pains of my life were rocked away.

In another session, Ed stood in front of me, with his back to me and bent forward at the waist. He carefully hoisted me up onto his torso so that I was lying face down draped across his wide back. My feet and hands were dangling and I was perfectly balanced. In that position, I felt fully supported, all my weight being borne by another. Again, Ed rocked me back and forth. The burdens of my life loosened and dropped away. Like the Aboriginal little sister in *Rabbit-Proof Fence*, who was carried by her thirteen-year-old sibling across hundreds of miles after their escape from a government boarding school, I felt like I was being carried home on the back of great love.

In another of Manfred's structures, we imagined ourselves as marionettes, being moved about by an unseen puppeteer. Afterward, Manfred talked about the experience of "being moved" by another, a phrase with obvious double meanings. I thought of surrender, of being willing to be moved by a power greater than myself. Ah, *this* is what it feels like! Manfred called it simply "grace."

Being the *mover* was also an experience of grace—surrendering to curiosity and creativity, to the other person's humanity, and to my own memories, associations, and lessons. After sculpting a partner with a soft and slender body, I recorded these reflections:

> Feeling someone else's warm body move under my
> hands is primal. Like holding my child when he was
> a baby. Limp. Losing fluids. As we were riding along a
> prairie highway miles from home. And the two of us, his
> parents, didn't understand a tiny baby's needs beyond
> what I'd learned from Dr. Spock. His crying was limp,
> too, and frightening, and my impatient husband also
> had to be soothed. Who holds us in such moments and
> strokes our hair? Let me stroke this one I am holding

now for all those times her babies were sick and she was frightened.

I found, in this Group Motion retreat, how pleasurable and healing it can be to move and to make sounds. I learned a lot about listening. To move with others, whether in a creative dance setting or in our day-to-day dance of living, requires pointed attentiveness to them. As Manfred often said, "The listening is done with touch, and the energy that is communicated in the touch is what brings about the movement." A feather-light touch, I learned, generates a different energy and response than a firm grip.

After returning home from the retreat, I found myself living more comfortably in my body and being kinder to it. For a time, everything seemed like a dance—moving into my chair in front of my computer, lifting a pan out of the oven, opening the mail. Everyone I encountered became my dance partner. When someone touched me, I "listened" and moved accordingly, even joining in a rhythmic flow with a friend as she helped me repair my dining room chairs.

Since we're always in our bodies and often moving about and making sounds, what a treasure it is to do these things consciously. Every movement, then, becomes a dance; every interchange, group motion.

𝕊 Chapter Sixteen

The Language of the Body Is Spoken Here

*M*ovement was our primary language when we were born. Then we learned words, and this native "tongue" was mostly silenced. What if, as adults, we again embraced this elemental mode of communicating that came to us so naturally? If we created more occasions to romp and play together, wouldn't we be more connected and creative? If we trusted and enjoyed the movement and messages of our bodies, wouldn't we take better care of them—and communicate more honestly and vibrantly? If we danced together with those unlike us, could we even perhaps reduce the chance of going to war?

From experiences such as the Group Motion retreat, I believe it's possible for us to learn, or relearn, these ways of communicating. Yet, many of us have become so used to suppressing our bodily expression that we also have a lot of unlearning to do.

Sometimes I feel like a prisoner in my body, especially when I'm sitting in a meeting or a class. Everyone just *sits* there. The only motion comes from the lips. At a conference I attended on adult learning, I was distressed by the lack of lively interaction. Even during the occasional small-group discussions, participants remained seated at the tables where they had been sitting for hours. Except during standard break and mealtime activity, no one moved throughout the entire seven-hour day.

After the first two hours of sit-and-listen, I was in pain. All of me had showed up for this event hungry for learning, but only my eyes, ears, and brains were fed. The rest of me starved and shriveled. The only muscles to get some exercise were those tensing up. Another participant, equally stressed by "sititis," bemoaned, "We *know* better than this."

America has become a nation of sitters, and this debilitating virus may be spreading along with the globalization of technology, threatening an international plague. We've not only been well-trained to sit still in order to learn (and the amount of time we need to spend learning keeps growing in our fast-changing world), but both work and leisure time are increasingly spent chair-bound in front of screens. We speak to, and are spoken to, by machines. Arrays of computers, video games, movies, television, and video and DVD players create altars from which the ministers of commerce and entertainment preach and sing to us about what we need to do to be savvy. Ironically, fitness and massage centers proliferate, offering a place to work off the stress and build up endurance for another day of sitting and fleshless interaction. At the same time, obesity is becoming epidemic, perhaps in part because our bodies crave action and touch; we reach for food so we can at least feel our jaws moving and experience some sensory pleasures.

Between break times at the conference, I found myself eyeing the food table repeatedly as the day droned on. I wasn't hungry but desperate for any excuse to get up and move, anything that would activate and soothe my stifled body. At one break, I cheer-led a few people around me in some stretching moves in order to survive the rest of the morning, but by lunchtime I had become too antsy from all that sitting and left the conference. While much good was accomplished at this event, in my mind it lacked the kind of vitality the conference was touting. Learning with only the mind is like eating only protein. The brain gets a temporary hit, but the body as a whole craves an energy boost. Attention span is limited, and what learning takes place feels lifeless.

I am sad that our cultural conditioning has profoundly suppressed the pleasure of living in and from our bodies. Yet I take a deeply satisfying, remembering breath when I read what Matthew Budd and Larry Rothstein describe in *You Are What You Say*: "Your body is the manifestation at this very moment of millions and millions of years of evolution. . . . Your body is precious, infinitely complex and brilliantly sensitive to environmental triggers. It is the vehicle of your awareness, of your activity, of your dignity and of your love." I don't ever want to forget this. I don't want to live into my old age with the magnificence of my body on hold.

Getting together in a group to learn something doesn't have to be a sitting marathon. I remember a conference I attended where bodies were given their due. I watched and "oohed" with delight as the opening session featured dancers sweeping down the aisles, unfurling lengthy swaths of blue cloth. As they reached the front, the dancers aligned the waving swaths side by side to create a rolling-river dance. The dancing, combined with music and story telling the life-giving history and promise of the Mississippi River, served to welcome participants to Minneapolis, which is situated near the headwaters of the great waterway. To my added delight, the dancers included not only the usual slender women with long, flowing hair but sprightly children and men with gray hair, including one with a hefty girth.

This opening celebration enveloped me and the thousand other people in attendance in a live expression of the conference's theme of creating a better, more inclusive world for all people. Not surprisingly, the conference also ended with a dance, bringing all the participants into a unifying spiral. In addition, many of the workshops I attended at the conference engaged attendees in activities that stimulated the senses and got us out of our chairs. I tarried after the closing session of this conference, not wanting to leave this climate of celebration and whole-being participation.

What if all learning experiences had this kind of vibrancy as the norm? I might have stayed a lot longer at the adult learning conference that I left early if the day had included more embodied learning opportunities. Perhaps the state demographer, when reporting on the aging of the state's population, could have had us stand up and take a step to the right for each percentage point that the average age of Minnesotans will increase in the next fifty years. Or he could have assigned us to decade groups and then had some of the people in a group shift into the next older group as he cited the shifting trends. Moving like that, I would have *felt* and *seen* the nature of these statistics, and remembered better what he said. I could also imagine a call-and-response singer to help reinforce other critical information at intervals throughout the day.

Even the small-group discussions would have been more invigorating had we done at least some of them standing up. Have you ever noticed how much more expressive people are when they're standing and talking? Arms and hands fly. High-fives happen. Even hips get in motion to accentuate a point. I once heard that if you want to get to know someone better, go walking with them: people are more honest when they're in motion. I think that's true. Chances are that we can be more creative when more of our body is engaged in the creative process. Not that we can't be vibrant and inventive when we're sitting, but trained as we have been from childhood to "sit down and be still," it takes extra effort.

Antonio Damasio, in *The Feeling of What Happens*, brings out another dimension of the body's magnificence, when he says, "All emotions use the body as their theater." What a fine show this truth promises, but unfortunately, the theatre of the body is often dark. Conditioned as we are to operate as talking heads, most of the marvel of our body is muted. We rein in its expression and choke off its voice. But emotions crave physical expression, and there is often mutiny when healthy means of doing so are denied. Getting high—on alcohol or drugs, compulsive eating or exercise—can become the substitute for genuine emotional vitality. Psychosomatic symptoms may appear. People may even get into violent fights, go on shooting rampages, or use other perverse forms of bodily expression. Yet, such destructive outlets for our feelings may be less appealing—or necessary—if we become attentive audience members to our body as theatre.

One couple told me that, on the verge of a familiar nasty argument, they decided to try a new approach. As frequent Group Motion participants, they decided to draw upon their creative dance experiences. Instead of engaging in the usual battle of words, they took turns showing each other through gestures and movement what pained them about thieir troubling issue. As they trusted their bodies to do the talking, both of them felt some deep-seated fears welling up beneath the anger—fears they hadn't been aware were there. In watching each other discover and reveal this hidden fright, their animosity dissipated. The other person was no longer seen as "wrong," but scared, vulnerable, in need of understanding and care. This experience in body honesty led them to compassion and greater acceptance.

Sometimes, in cases of physical danger, we may need to communicate with physical force, or at least be prepared to do so. Years ago I took a basic self-defense course for women so I could feel more confident if I were ever assaulted. I learned to thrust my fist forward from a balanced and forceful posture. I learned how to stomp on an attacker's foot and kick at his knee. Part of what gave these moves force was combining them with a sharp, belly-based yell—"Hah!" Later, I changed the exclamation to "No!" which felt even more powerful.

While I've never been in a physical confrontation where I needed to use these practices, they fortify me for a variety of situations that seem dangerous or challenging. When I anticipate a difficult meeting with someone, especially when my confidence is fragile, I sometimes practice a few self-defense moves before leaving home. I could simply try to talk myself into feeling confident, of course, but I find it easier to get to that state if I first take a stand for myself physically. When my whole body is thrusting forward, well supported, I shed my self-doubts. I'm not holding my breath or holding back. I'm putting myself out there, all of me.

This preparation, while garnering fortitude, does not, however, make me confrontational or defensive. In fact, the act of ardently expressing "no" several times during my warm-up at home tends to get any hostile feelings out of my system so I don't carry them into the meeting. Instead, I enter the meeting feeling strong, clear, capable, calm. I use my full voice, and my whole body is more expressive than usual. I'm not threatening, but I'm *there*. Authentic, integrated body language declares a presence and supports statements of truth. And there is safety in truth—for everyone involved.

Once I took a part-time job to supplement my income. During the orientation, my boss, whom I had judged to be a sensitive and thoughtful person, referred to his employees (all women) as "the girls." I was stunned to hear this demeaning language still being used, and I barely heard anything else the man said. I walked out of the session bristling. When I got home, a few "no" thrusts focused my anger into a clarifying force. No longer fuming, I made an appointment with my new boss to express my concern. I was able to give him feedback about what he said in such a way that he thanked me for it.

When I returned home from the Group Motion retreat, I could hardly wait to dance again. Friends urged me to lead a few improvisational sessions and share with them some of Manfred's novel structures. Since then a group of us has continued to meet each Friday morning, using recorded rather than live music. Right from the beginning, I decided to participate in the movements as well as calling out the instructions for the dance. I simply had to. While drawing on Manfred's work, it wasn't long before I was also creating and leading simple and evocative movement structures of my own. Others in the group also sometimes suggested movement forms. In some sessions, we let nothing but the music be our guide. We just move as we are *moved*.

In fact, that would describe all the dancing. I may give some general direction—"Move lightly," "Let your movements be circular," "Move like you had nowhere to go"—but we each take great latitude in shaping that suggestion into a form. The "circular" movements may be someone's arms swinging around at her sides, or someone's whole body swirling in big swoops, or someone's feet rotating as she lies on her back.

Sooner or later, we always end up intersecting, moving in communication with one another. We bend, leap, and roll among each other, becoming, as one member put it, "bodies cooperating." The choreography is collaborative. Each of us creates forms from our internal impetus—the brushing, intertwining, and cradling of each other's heads, arms and hands, torsos, legs and feet. We can spend anywhere from a few minutes to an hour playing with a hundred ways of letting our hands be in conversation or folding ourselves over and around each other with childlike ease. We lose ourselves in getting to know the beauty and touch of our bodies in motion.

Sometimes we make faces, telling our stories with all forty-five muscles. We are giving witness to what theologian and philosopher Thomas Moore, in *Care of the Soul*, says about the face being "a map of the soul." Drooped eyes, wrinkled brows, a wide grin, or sunken cheeks are markers of spirit. During our dance sessions, our faces have a chance to expand into full repertoire and reveal both well-marked and subtle terrains.

I look over at Cathy, a lithe, tiny-bodied woman with long, coal-black curls. She dances a few feet in front of me and I see her jaws stretched wide open, cheeks pulled up and back, nose crinkled, and eyebrows raised. This scream pose, held and exaggerated, is not hers alone. In it, I am meeting the face of terror centuries old. I have worn it myself when my childhood teddy bear was yanked away from me by my teasing brother, when the precious certainty of my marriage shattered, when a friend I counted on said our friendship was over. Cathy holds this pose on her face until the terror it speaks has had its full say. Then, gradually, her face remolds and I see bared teeth, set jaw, and slitted eyes. This time I am witnessing rage—hers, but also a rage I have known myself and that many others have known.

As I watch Cathy, I feel my face changing shape, too, sometimes in response to hers or the other dancers', sometimes displaying my own disappointments, desperation, exhilaration, or an array of other emotions. Over a short time, drama after drama is staged by each of us, climaxes and denouements are reached, curtains are closed. Comedies get equal time, and sometimes giggles overcome us; we roll around like preschoolers and end up collapsing in a puppy pile.

One morning just two of us showed up and our haggard faces declared "What a week!" I was tempted to ask the other woman why she was so distressed and to fill her in on my difficulties of the week. But I feared we'd dispel the magic of our dancing time and become more agitated than relieved from talking about the week's dramas. I suggested instead that we create a "newscast," each "reporting" to the other on the happenings of her week through movement.

After our usual warm-up stretching, I began the newscast by reporting "live" from a "crime scene." My pounding arms and stomping feet showed that I felt like pouncing on someone whose behavior had riled me that week. For the next "news" item, my body began heaving back and forth in wailing motions, telling of the grief I felt over my long-loved piano going out the door to a new home.

The news dance continued, weaving together from my week more moments of confusion, loneliness, regret, and sadness, but also joy. The energy of each experience burst out through my torso, limbs, neck, and head. The dance became my journal embodied. When it ended, with me on my knees, my arms folded loosely across my chest, and my torso in a sustained rocking motion, I felt like I had been in labor. At last I had given birth to my week's story, full-sized and healthy. My experience became flesh, with another dancer as midwife and witness. My distress and delights were reborn into a flowing, wordless form that illuminated my experience as sacred story.

In a later session, we did the newscast dance again, and after each person finished her story, the rest of us danced a response to it. No words were adequate in the presence of the newborn story, and none were needed. The language of movement mirrored and magnified this infant, and nourished it like mother's milk. And the birth-giving multiplied. More life was generated within the responding dancers in forms of circling and rocking arms, blessing strokes, leaps of triumph, and other creations.

These were "knowing" dances. When the others danced a response to my story in motion, I felt known. They had heard me. They *got* it. And I knew my own story more fully, from what my own body, as storyteller, revealed and from watching what my movements inspired in others. I found a hint of sweetness in what had only tasted bitter to me. I recognized a rage I had shrouded in silliness. And like all stories, once told, this story was no longer mine alone. It had a life of its own. It became a drop in the sea of stories from which all becomes known.

Every day we attempt to communicate and learn, mostly using words. But since our bodies are, by far, the biggest conveyors of our communication, perhaps we could give them the lead more often. What if we came to appreciate and expand the body's vocabulary and employed its finest grammar and syntax? In my Toastmasters meetings, we are often reminded to use gestures and facial expressions to help convey our message—the most elementary use of the body for effective communication. But there is so much more available if, rather than just *using* our bodies to communicate, we come to know the language of our bodies intimately and let it spill forth with ease.

Dances of the Heart

A little woman with nervous hair glanced at her hands. The man sitting across from her in the circle leaned forward on his cane, waiting. When he turned his face to mine, I saw an old shy smile, still fresh from boyhood but only at half-mast on one side. Next to him was a short, roundish woman all in purple, hat included. She was the liveliest in the group of a dozen people in their seventies and eighties gathered in a cluttered meeting room of the Southwest Senior Center, a small, storefront facility in an old Minneapolis neighborhood. They had come to dance and I was invited into their circle for the day.

For this dance, no one had to stand. Not that anyone there couldn't stand—at least with help; they just didn't do it any more than necessary. Whether from heavy weight, heavy spirits, fragile bones, or pure habit, they relied on the security of their chairs. Most were staring into space until dance leader Maria Genné arrived. A flurry of good mornings and out-of-breath unpacking of CDs from her bulky bag were complemented by sparkly greetings from other dance company members there to help her.

Maria is the artistic director of Kairos Dance Theatre, a Minneapolis-based, intergenerational company that works in senior centers, adult day care centers, schools, and other settings to create community dance experiences. From what she had told me, her work at Southwest exemplified my passion—

full-bodied living throughout our older years regardless of our "condition." Most of the people in this group had physical limitations. Some had a history of social isolation and depression. I had asked Maria if I could come and observe what happened when she got them dancing.

As Maria and her colleagues were setting up for the morning activities, no one in the circle spoke much. I thought of how small children sitting in their places before class would be talking and wiggling and tossing things, and the teacher would have to quiet them down to begin. Here were old ones, perhaps long ago well trained to sit still and be quiet, and perhaps further silenced in this time of their life by the effects of illness, boredom, or even despair. What is there to say when you live alone in a high-rise, with windows on just one side of your tiny apartment and rarely a visitor?

When words are scarce, bodies can do the talking. Maria introduced the Name Game. Everyone in the room, including me, was invited to participate as Maria gave the reminder instructions for the opening ritual: "Say your name, tell us how you're feeling, and then show us your feeling through a gesture."

First to speak up was the woman in purple. "I'm Janie, and I'm not feeling so good today. Got a little cold. So . . ."—she paused to set up her summation words—"I'm tired." With the word "tired," her body sagged forward and she heaved a sigh. Everyone in the circle became her mirror, saying, "Janie. Tired," as our bodies sagged and sighed in response. Next was the half-smile man. His speech was slow, words hard to form. "I'm Melvin. I'm glad to see you." He was grinning at Maria. One hand extended a gesture of welcome. The group responded with "Melvin. Glad to see you," echoing his hand movement. Next was Leah, who was "excited," arms thrusting up in the air. Not all the arms in the room rose as high in response, but all moved upward.

And so it went around the room, each person going from

a mere chair occupier to being known and appreciated. Smiles filled every face.

A light calypso beat came from the CD player and the next round of dancing began. We all turned our chairs to face a partner for the mirror game. We were instructed to move in ways that were enjoyable, and to take turns "mirroring" each other's movements. One partner was designated blue, one red. The reds began. Hands, arms, head, and in some cases, the whole upper body started to move in time to the music. Simple, slow movements—hands waving back and forth, shoulders moving in circles, whatever each body might find pleasure in. Some of the dancers contained their expression within a few inches, others swayed and stretched widely. "Blues" followed as best they could, keeping a close eye on their partners' moves. My "blue" partner, Henry, was in a wheelchair. His arms appeared lax, unaccustomed to much activity. As I danced, his mirroring movements were erratic and jerky, but his eyes concentrated on my every move. When it was Henry's turn to be red, he leaned forward and a wide grin emerged. His thick, gnarled hands took the lead, making vigorous moves only half under his control. I was so taken by how he was leaning into life, despite his limitations, that I had trouble concentrating on his movements.

From there, we did a tossing game—lofting imaginary objects back and forth across the circle. Mimes of a ball, a hat, a "hot potato" being thrown and caught brought forth choruses of "oohs" and a roomful of bright eyes and laughter.

From there it wasn't hard for Maria to move the group into practice for their "Dances of the Heart" performance scheduled for Valentine's Day at an elementary school. The movements had been choreographed during the weeks this group had met, and each movement represented a memory, a feeling, a story of one of the members—hands clasped over the heart to express Dorothy's sorrow over her dead husband, a baby-holding gesture for Alphie's new great-granddaughter, a stretch upward in celebration of Janie's improved health.

All this without ever getting out of their chairs!

Finally, Maria brought out a parachute. Tucked into its bag, it had seemed small, lifeless, insignificant, not unlike the people around the circle whose full capacity could easily go unrealized and unseen if not for this time of dancing together. Spread open, the enormous white flowing cloth filled the circle space, lacking only a lifting movement to billow into fullness. Everyone grabbed an edge. As the parachute was raised in unison, it rounded above us, almost taking us up with it; then it dropped, floating slowly downward in waves that gently swept us along. Up and down, up and down, over and over. We were flying; we were floating. Every *body* was alive!

Arms that had barely moved above the waist before were now stretching high. "Tired" Janie was up on her feet, and so was almost everyone else. Smiles were wide. "Woooo! Wow!" Big bright orange and blue balls were tossed on top of the waving, billowing cloth and rolled recklessly about. When they rolled toward someone in the circle, gleeful squeals erupted as that person swooped up the cloth to redirect the balls up in the air or across the cloth to someone else. This was play. This was exercise. This was community. This was ecstasy.

While some might label this group of people as old, weak, and uninteresting, what their bodies had to say in our time together had endeared them to me. I came to know them as vibrant, creative, caring people. This was not dance as performance—though it would also become that—it was dance as experience. We were all dancing our lives.

Part Four

Some Body's Left

Who knows when we're going to be sick—
real sick. It could happen any minute. Our
bodies are working fine. We're walking, talking, laughing, doing dishes, driving to the
store, and then there's a twinge, a blur, a
numbness we feel only for a second. Or longer. It's nothing. It's the start of something.
It passes, like a thousand other twinges and
blurs and numb feelings, but it's not over. It
comes back. It happens again. Or maybe it
doesn't pass, and the twinge tightens, bending us into a pretzel, and we live with ice
packs and go for treatment after treatment
until it's better. And then we forget it. Or the
blur intensifies and there's a dizziness and a
pain in the colon, and it finally takes a Mayo
doctor to say, though it might be a virus,
they'd have to run more tests. Or it becomes
cancer and we lose a leg like dancer Homer
Avila did, and become determined, like he
did, to continue dancing, finding new ways
to move without losing balance.

Bodies in Pain

I've long resisted the image of old age as a period of vegetation in a nursing home. My eye instead is on the centenarians still going to work every day or still tending their gardens. I want to stay healthy and active like them until shortly before I die. That's the natural process of aging according to contemporary science—to keep functioning quite nicely until the year or so preceding death. Diseases commonly associated with aging, such as heart disease and dementia, don't actually result from the aging process itself but from genetic, lifestyle, and environmental influences. So there's nothing that says I automatically have to "go downhill" as I get older.

Yet, like many other people looking ahead to older years, I have some fears about ill health. Whenever my body hurts or functions poorly, I wonder, *Will this condition become chronic? Will it be debilitating?* I'm aware that seeping underground in the back acres of my mind is the question I most fear: *Is this a precursor to death?*

My hands have been swelling slightly for several years. The swelling was no more than a nuisance, so I mostly ignored it for a long time. Though my rings no longer moved easily over the joints, I could get them on and off with the help of hand lotion. But when someone grabbed my hand in an overly friendly squeeze, I winced. And knocking my swollen knuckles on someone's door had become a painful exercise.

It's probably just an allergic reaction to something I'm eating, I kept thinking, since I was also having some vague digestive problems. So I tried to notice when the swelling worsened and what I'd eaten that day, but I couldn't find the culprit.

After several years of puzzlement, I decided it was time to get a medical opinion. The nurse practitioner on duty gave my hands a brief look. "Oh, you've got arthritis," she declared matter-of-factly, as if saying I had a cold.

Her words hit me like a bullhorn blast, slapped me tight against the back of my chair, and snapped me into mild shock. *Arthritis. Arthritis.* The word seemed long and loud as it echoed like a death knell throughout my brain. "All of us get it sooner or later," the nurse went on, with a "too bad" shake of her head and a pensive glance at her own hands. Inside my skull, "arthritis" tolled, accompanied by "lifelong," "no cure," "old age," and similar themes I had long heard associated with the disease.

Breaking into my somber mental racket, the nurse spoke again. "What kind of work do you do?"

I could barely reply, "I'm a writer."

"That'll do it," she responded. "All that repetitive activity . . ."

A mix of sadness and low-level panic settled into my nervous system. I sat motionless, like a rabbit hearing the bark of a dog. Frantic and fatalistic thoughts demanded my attention: *So this is what all those years of keyboarding have brought me to? Is this my legacy for being a writer?* I had flashing images of the times I pushed on with my writing for hours and hours, without taking breaks. I recalled the hand-stretching exercises I had learned to keep my hands agile, but had neglected. I pictured the ergonomically correct keyboards I never thought I could afford, or get used to. *I didn't think it would come to this. This can't be happening. I've just been doing what I love. I take very good care of my health usually—a lot better than most people. This isn't fair!*

Gnarled hands I had seen in nursing homes appeared like snapshots in my brain. I felt my jaw slackening, my forehead wrinkling, my shoulders slumping. *Is this where I'm headed? Will I have to give up my writing? Should I cut back immediately so my hands don't get worse? But who will I be without my hands? They are my voice! They are my survival. Without them, how can I even make a living?*

Even in the midst of my panic, my reaction struck me as extreme, foolish. I knew that lots of people have arthritis and simply live with it. My mother did. Yet, this revelation of a chronic and progressive condition stung me as the first major personal harbinger of the dreaded going downhill. And I had indeed known people for whom arthritis was extremely painful and debilitating. As I thought of them, a flood of worst-case scenarios slipped me further into survival mode. *My God, will I become so crippled that I can't turn keys in the door or dress myself or even stand up without pain? How will I manage? Who will take care of me?*

The nurse's voice interjected into my thoughts, "Here's a prescription for the pain. Just take it as needed."

Another startle response. *Pain! There's going to be pain?* I remember the despondent complaints and wincing faces of people I've known with arthritis.

But she doesn't understand. I never said anything about pain. I barely even feel any pain in my hands. Sure, the swelling is a little uncomfortable, but I don't need any medication for pain, thank you very much.

But here she's giving me the prescription as if "pain" is inevitable. That must be my fate.

Getting diagnosed with a chronic condition happens every day to millions of people, especially the old. We want to know what's "wrong" with our bodies, and we look to someone trained in body sciences to tell us. We hope for a quick fix. Sometimes we get it, but sometimes the disease has no cure. We are left to live with a life sentence. Things are never the same. We can't be expected to like it. We may even refuse to believe it. No one, at least no one I know, wants to have their wings clipped.

After the diagnosis, we search for solutions. Some people rush around for second opinions, look for cures in far-away places, try complementary approaches ranging from supplements to aromatherapy to colon cleansing. Then, there's positive thinking, hands-on healing, prayer, and downright stubbornness. I've taken my turn at all of the above. We're all looking for a way to take charge and get answers, and if that doesn't work, then a miracle will do nicely. We want to be well. It's instinctual. It makes sense.

But we don't always get what we want. We may be left with a troubling permanent condition. At first, we speak of "my arthritis" or "my heart problem" in the same way we speak of "my in-laws," foreigners of sorts with whom we must try to get along as best we can. Before long, our condition merges with our self-definition. When asked, "How are you?" we respond with, "Well, my arthritis is . . . ," followed by an update on whether the condition has gotten better or worse. The in-laws have moved in under our roof. We wish they'd leave, but we claim them as our own anyway—our cross to bear.

Welcome, anger, my friend. Welcome, fear. That's how Thich Nhat Hanh recommends we greet our troubling emotions. Welcome them in as guests, he says. Make friends with them. Treat them honorably. Let them have their say. I wonder if the same approach makes sense for our physical troubles. They, too, are visitors. What if we welcomed them, got to know them, listened to their stories?

That sounds noble, but hard. We have our hands plenty full already coping with the strains of the illness. There is not only the physical discomfort, but the treatments and side effects, and maybe even loss of skills and the need to move to more accommodating living arrangements. We also have to face the responses of those around us. Especially for people in their later years, illness equals "old" and pathetic in the public eye. It arouses the leprosy response. Who wants to be around someone like that? Few people rush to visit nursing homes or pay a call on someone wincing with pain and dulled by medication.

Maybe it's asking too much to welcome illness with open arms. Perhaps the most that can be hoped for is moment-by-moment attentiveness. *What is happening now, at this moment?* In fact, that may be what the Buddhist monk means by welcoming.

I remember with fondness the evening Jim and Shelby Andress attended a dinner party at my home. Shelby had been a friend and business colleague for close to a year, but this was the first time I had met her husband. Jim had Alzheimer's. Over the dozen years or so since the condition was first diagnosed, the two of them had decided to share intimately with each other—and with many others—their experience of how the disease affected each of them as it progressed. They even gave talks and media interviews on their experience (including an appearance on *Oprah*).

In meetings I had attended with Shelby as we worked together on a project, she often told me of the anguish and awe that surfaced as she and Jim faced each new loss together. Each story felt to me like a revelation of her heart, deliberately given as a gift. She told how one morning Jim tried to dress himself, and his sleeves and buttons were all in the wrong places. Shelby smiled at him in exasperation and said, "Jim, you are a case!" His characteristic humor came through in his reply, "You should have known me when I wore a suit. Then you would have called me a 'suitcase.'"

As the months and years wore on, his increasingly rare lucid moments often brought tender and surprising comments. He would tell her he understood how hard this was for her and how much he appreciated what she was doing. He would talk about the need for their spirits to stay in touch after he lost all his mental abilities and also after he died. When he felt himself disconnecting more and more from reality, he talked to Shelby about feeling like a "balloon bouncing around with a broken string."

At the time of the dinner party, Jim was still conversing in near-normal manner some of the time. He arrived wearing a pleasant smile and offering his hand in greeting. At the dinner table, though, I watched Shelby matter-of-factly put a bib on Jim, cut up and put his food on the fork for him, and occasionally lift a cup to his lips, each time checking with him first about whether this is what he wanted. Each time, he took a moment to consider, and said yes. These exchanges struck me as acts of reverence.

Despite his physical limitations, Jim talked freely and alertly with the ten other people at the table, contributing insights from his years of experience in education. His speech was a bit slow and halting at times, but his ideas clear for the most part. Once, however, well into a lengthy commentary that commanded everyone's attention, he stopped midsentence, obviously unable to find the next thought. Aware of everyone's discomfort with the long pause, he finally smiled and mused, "Now, this is awkward, isn't it?" sparking laughter as he graciously put us all at ease.

Shelby never stepped in unnecessarily to rescue him. Her respect for him, and his for her, were palpable. When the activity of the dinner tired him, she unobtrusively helped him to a nearby recliner, where he could rest within earshot of the continuing conversation.

What I witnessed that evening was a tender love story, and also a profound lesson in mindful living. Both Jim and Shelby showed, moment by moment, a willingness to accept each loss, each difficulty, each tender moment with grace, humor, and full attention to their emotions. Together they tended to Jim's needs and the changes in his body in a sacred manner, as if nothing more important could be happening at that moment for either of them. I can imagine the washing of Jesus' feet by Mary Magdalene having that same quality.

Alzheimer's, diabetes, heart disease, and other names for illnesses are medical descriptions for a set of symptoms, but they do not describe what is happening for the sick individual. Every illness shows up in specific physical experiences, giving us an opportunity to bear witness and respond mindfully as Jim and Shelby did. My experience of arthritis is tightness along my fingers and difficulty in curling my hand. It is the struggle with putting my rings on and taking them off. It is the pain when rapping on a door or trying to open a sealed jar lid. It is also an assortment of other minute activities going on within my body, changes in body chemistry and energy flow and other dynamics that I haven't yet learned how to notice and name.

A mindful response for Jim was allowing Shelby to tie on a bib to catch the spills resulting from his poor self-feeding skills. In my case, with my arthritis, it might be to ask someone else to open the jar. This is respectful attention to the immediate, practical body needs of the moment.

There are also opportunities for another kind of attention. Thomas Moore, in *Care of the Soul*, says that our body "has some link with consciousness and a particular mode of expression." He refers to a contention by Freud's colleague Sandor Ferenczi, that "body parts [have] their own 'organ eroticism.'" In commenting on Ferenczi's notion, Moore says, "As I understand him, he meant that each organ has its own private life and, you might say, personality that takes pleasure in its activities. [If] my colon was unhappy, and if I could attend to its complaint I might begin to understand what was making it uneasy, or, so to speak, 'dis-easy.'"

We are hungry to find meaning in illness. Always people ask, why is this happening? In our efforts to play close attention to the "private life" of our body, we may never come up with a precise logical link that clarifies the cause of an illness. Yet, it is a logical place to look for what may be less clear but more important—its story, its music, its nature. What will it teach us? How might it please us or awaken us?

"The body is the soul presented in its richest and most expressive form," says Moore, and he also calls it "an immense source of imagination." James Hillman, too, refers to the body as "a citadel of metaphors" when we are aging. Might the slowing of our body awaken us to the value of moving more slowly? Might viewing our wrinkles in the mirror reveal something about honesty and ultimate vulnerability? Hillman says that "it is an enormous mistake to read the phenomena of later life as an indication of death rather than as initiations into another way of life."

John, a man in his fifties with bulky, rounded shoulders, came in great pain to a workshop I co-led on the wisdom of the aging body. He told me that he had been experiencing back problems for some time. In the workshop, we did an exercise developed by Sam Keen, in which participants closed their eyes and took several steps backward, imagining and attempting to re-experience with each step how it felt to be different personal ancestors back through several generations.

John was eager to talk when we gathered in a circle for discussion after the exercise. He said, "I could really feel how hard it was for my father and his father before him. I came from a family of miners and they worked extremely hard. During the exercise, I could recognize how burdened I have felt. It's as if I'm carrying the same burdens they carried on my back."

My co-presenter, Brian Brooks, asked John to arrange Brian's body into a shape that represented this sense of burden that John felt. John responded by bending Brian over at the waist until Brian's torso was leaning forward, parallel to the floor. He extended Brian's right arm forward into a reaching motion, and bent the left arm so it stretched backward, with the elbow jutting out to the side.

"Yes, that's exactly it," John exclaimed, excited by his creation. "That's exactly how it feels. It's like I'm carrying this heavy weight on my back all the time.

"The men before me were used to bending down to go into the mine. That must be how they felt about life. You had to bend down and go to work and there was no way out. And that's the way I've been feeling in my life, like it's all hard work, like it's this huge burden. No wonder I have back problems. I remember my dad and my uncle walking around bent over. And now I'm doing the same thing."

Once John came to recognize the story he carried in his body, he could begin to rewrite it. John eagerly re-sculpted Brian into a man standing tall, shoulders in proper alignment, neck long, head upright. When John took a step back to view his creation, I noticed that he, too, was standing in that position.

"How do you react when you see that?" I asked John, pointing to Brian.

"I feel free," he said, throwing his hands up in the air. "I feel free."

Pain, disability, and illness, whether chronic or temporary, change us. They make us stop and take notice. When any of these conditions happens to me, my first response is generally a deeply conditioned one. I want it to stop it as fast as possible. But I am reminded by John's experience that, whether or not I find a cure, or even relief, a higher level of healing may come if I regard my body as storyteller and listen closely.

I woke up very groggy one Thursday morning. In fact, I had been feeling groggy for two days, and a flare-up of my occasional low-back pain added to the discomfort. Working at a client's office that day, I couldn't seem to concentrate. When the day's work was over, I wanted to go home and lie down, but I had told a friend with several serious health problems I would visit her. When I arrived at her apartment, she was depressed and lethargic. With my low energy, I was glad to sink into the couch next to her. I did my best to comfort her and gave her a foot massage. After a while, I prompted her to go for a short walk, hoping that would perk us both up. I was shivering, but attributed this to the chilly, damp weather. I could hardly wait to get home, and just getting my clothes off to get into bed seemed like a labor. I was asleep within minutes after nine o'clock.

By midnight, I had made two bathroom trips, and I could tell my sweatiness was more than the usual hot flashes. I took my temperature; it read 101°F. I almost felt relief. No wonder I had been so weary! Assuming I had the flu, I braced myself for a few days of misery.

The next day my whole body ached as if I had been beaten, and my temperature hovered near 103°F. Two days later, I began to panic. The fever and aching had intensified. My bedclothes and bedding were soaked with sweat at night, and my body shivered off and on during the day. Except for a brief "It's just a virus" doctor visit, I'd been by myself for three days. What if this goes on much longer? What if I run out of food? Will there be anyone to help me? My son lives a hour or more away by bus and doesn't have a car. My friends have busy lives and live in other parts of the city. I didn't want to bother them, and in my anguished state, I started to find fault with living by myself, for not having done more to make friends with my neighbors, for not having enough friends. I felt terribly alone and increasingly desperate.

Then, on Sunday evening, I dragged myself outside to sit on

my front step. I was craving sunlight, looking for a sign of hope. As I sat there, I noticed a large rash on the back of my left leg. When I looked closer, I saw it was in the shape of a bull's-eye—a sure sign of Lyme disease. A sharp cry escaped my lips. Despite the many warnings I had read about doing skin checks for the Lyme-carrying deer ticks when in Minnesota's northern woods, I realized I hadn't done so after a recent stay there.

I remembered a man I once knew who had this diagnosis. His whole life was shattered. He could no longer work, he lived with a great deal of pain, and he had to rely on others to take care of much of his household and personal business. I had pitied him. Now I assumed this would be my fate. I imagined my whole life suddenly being sucked into a black hole. I felt the urge to cry, but my tear ducts must have been too weary to open up. The heat of the sun intensified my sweating, but I could not move back inside my house for a long time.

The next day a doctor reassured me that, since the disease was caught early, an antibiotic would cure it. Somehow I couldn't believe him. I had never heard of a cure before—only many terrible warnings about this dreaded condition. Besides, I didn't like this doctor. He seemed too eager, as if he were trying to cover up something, or just trying to make me feel better.

To make matters worse, the antibiotic effects didn't start for two more days. My temperature eventually reached 105°F and I feared I would lose my mind. At one point, as I got up from my couch to put a fresh cool cloth on my forehead, I had a strange thought: I wondered if I could be happy in this debilitated state. I had just read a book that said we can find happiness in every situation. Most people aren't happy because they don't intend to be, the book said. Intention is key. I decided it was worth trying. If I could be happy under these circumstances, then overlooking everyday inconveniences like running out of bread or getting telemarketing calls would be a snap. I became willing to listen to my body instead of despairing about it. Could it, I wondered, in this experience of illness, hold a salvation story that I was missing because I was so caught up in feeling crucified?

Lying around for almost a week, unable to live my ordinary life, I already had been noticing my body much of the time. I was paying attention to what was wrong with it and trying to get it to feel better. Now I began to pay attention in a different way.

I feel like such a blob, a weighted piece of body mass sprawled here on the couch. I can barely get myself to and from the bathroom and the refrigerator. I am, however, breathing. Every few seconds I feel my chest lift and lower in an easy, constant rhythm. I hear the brushing of air against the inside surface of my nostrils, glad for the coolness as it enters, relieved by the discharge of heat as it leaves. I notice a tiny throbbing inside my chest. It is my faithful heart, keeping me alive. Muscles in my face are slack. There is none of the usual scrunching of the forehead; I'm not straining to figure out anything. Jaw and tongue rest; I have no need or energy to form words, or to hold them back. Hands and arms lie limp; no internal parental voice tells them to get busy. Shoulders and back are relaxed; no state of vigilant readiness is necessary to respond to what life might demand next.

This pervasive state of relaxation feels unfamiliar. I cannot work. I cannot do for others. I cannot perform or impress any-one with my knowledge, my words, or my cleverness. I cannot muster my usual hurry up and get things done mode. No effort is possible. No effort is required. No effort is . . . effortless.

Here I am, then, just breathing, feeling the thumping of my heart, appreciating. Isn't this what I've been wanting—to live in each moment with more ease, less effort, and more gratitude? Haven't I wanted to live without the constant feeling of pres-sure to perform, to succeed, to make a living, to get someone to notice and want what I have to offer? Right now, no one is wanting anything of me. I'm not expecting anything of myself either. So this is how it feels to just be? Not the fever and the achiness, of course, but the unagitated sense of no demands, no need to do. I am "hangin' out" again, this time not in a dance workshop. It is my given state of being.

This may be my daily dance for a long, long time, this state of just being. It's possible, despite what the doctor says, that I won't get better or be able to do any more than I can do right now. This may be my new life. If it is, nearly all the things I now think of as making up "me" and my life would dissolve. No more being known as a speaker and workshop leader. No more creating with words and receiving notes in the mail telling me how helpful they have been. No more going to plays, classes, conferences, parties, or parks. Perhaps no more ability even to cook my meals or clean my house. And no more need to do any of this. My life could be like that from now on.

How will I live, then? How will I meet expenses? I know I'll be taken care of somehow. Disability support from Social Security, maybe? But that's surely not enough to live on. And I won't be able to take care of my home. Oh, I hope I don't have to give up my home, this beautiful place I'm so fond of. But yes, I may have to leave it for someplace where sick people are cared for. Will it come down to that, living in a room somewhere, with someone looking in on me from time to time? If it does, when everything else is taken away, I will still be at home in my breathing, flesh-covered body.

I gaze down across my torso and limbs as if examining a new-born or an old woman stretched out on a hospital bed. Look at the thin, creviced walls of skin, full of bumps and oddly shaped. Look at the flattened breasts, loosely arranged across my chest. Look at the domed belly, smooth and evenly expanding with each breath. Look at the long fingers, curled out of habit. Look at the red and blue rivers bulging in jagged courses across my thighs. How large the feet, with nails in need of clipping. This has been my one faithful home all my life. It will do nicely for the duration.

I imagine standing to the side and lifting my body, like picking up a baby or a sickly person nearing death, just to hold and wonder at this fragile being. I think of when I was sitting next to my sister for a few days during her final weeks, after traveling the three hundred miles from my home to visit her. With her insides rapidly being devoured by cancer, she was little more than bloated flesh. Yet, she was flesh, and her presence blessed me.

As others tended to the needs of her body, I sat with her, to love her, to breathe with her as long as I could. Her every sigh or shift of limb interested me. Had I never noticed before how she moved, how her cheeks were rounded, how long were her legs? I think I missed knowing her body, except when looking for clues about how she regarded me—a raised eyebrow, an approving smile, a firming up of the jaw. Now, there she lay, this woman so resembling me in appearance and vocal quality that I was once mistaken for her by her close friends.

In many ways, my life, my character, and even my body were markedly shaped by the influence of my sister Lucille. She was the religious, disciplinarian older sister whose job was to turn me into a good girl. She herself was the ultimate good girl, becoming a hardworking, by-the-book Catholic nun. She even stayed the course when so many of her "sisters" left the convent and eventually became a school principal known for her dedication and firmness. I was only five years old when she left home to pledge her life to God's service. She was given the name Sister Patricia Ann; I grew up calling her Sister Pat. I barely remember her from my preschool years, yet I'm aware how much I was molded by her. As a young teen, she helped my mother, overburdened with nine children, to raise me. Over all the years we were separated, I continued to feel the imprint of her early guiding hand on my shoulder.

I became a good girl, too, obeying the rules and faithfully

tucking my true feelings and desires into tense jaw, shoulders, hips, and other pseudo-safe places. As with her, my ingratiating smile over a stern demeanor and my hard-work ethic were, for so many years, what I thought I needed in order to be pleasing, to be loved, to get it "right." The remnants of these character formations still shape me today.

For both of us, these rigid holding patterns often drove people away. A few years after my sister's death, when I met one of her religious sisters with whom she had lived and taught for many years, I understood when she told me Sister Pat had been hard to live with. That wasn't the whole story of who my sister was, of course. There were former students and others who knew her throughout the years who held her in high regard. But I understood, from my own experience, why she developed some of the body states she did, including the tightness of jaw that led to temporal mandibular joint (TMJ). Like her, all too often I have overused my jaw to hold back anger or to maintain an unwavering stance or a scolding hold.

As her pretensions and controlling ways were stripped away by illness and dependency, her body developed a softer quality. Her smile seemed more genuine. The furrowed-brow "scold" was gone. Her jaw seemed at ease.

This "new" body reflected the alchemic effect that illness had on her. The work-driven principal who had been in charge of a school and who had tried to control a whole lot more was no longer on duty. The God whom she had worked so hard to serve entered her heart most fully when surrender became her agenda. In the course of her illness, she became more open to love—both the giving and receiving of it. In her body's giving out, my sister found a deep love which her friends repeatedly said was so powerful that they were drawn to spend time with her over and over. I felt it, too, as I sat by her side.

During her third year of cancer, just a few months before her death, Sister Pat told a group of seminarians, "I feel with all my heart that I have lived my life more truly in these last two years than . . . in all the hard work I did before that. I was a workaholic and thought I was doing so much. . . . I came to the point where I couldn't work, couldn't do things. And I have found the Lord comes in marvelous ways and does marvelous things." She also told them, "I sit back amazed when people come up and say you have done so much for me and I say I didn't do anything. All I did was talk, and answer your questions. And sometimes not even that. What Our Lord did I don't know in these cases, but I have found His power so strong since I've been weak."

And near the end of her days, Sister Pat wrote in her prayer journal, "I thank you for the way you have used me to touch others, for the affirmation of your love. . . . Why does it take so long to see the value of people? Of love over things and activities?" These words confirmed what she said to me in our last conversation before the cancer overtook her brain. I remember asking her what she thought about as she looked back over her life. Her reply penetrated deep into my mind and heart: "I only wish I had learned to love sooner."

As I sat watching her breathe during my final visit, I wondered, Is this how it will be in the end for me—tensions worn down, shapes softened, ragged as the Velveteen Rabbit? Will I spend years, as she did, ravaged by disease's agony and depletion? Will I, too, be dependent on others to move me, feed me, wipe my bottom? As with her, will all my roles and accomplishments shrivel in significance and my only real home be a body bereft of ability? Will I have learned to love? I dream of completing my life like Meridel Le Sueur, with manuscripts strewn across my bed. Or like my Toastmaster friend Cookie Packer, who, shuffling down the hallway of the nursing home, visited other patients to make them laugh even when in great pain herself. But every body has its own story, in living and in dying.

⟿

As I lay on the couch, feverish with Lyme disease, I was not dying. But the quieting of my body had cooled the fevered fierceness of my life. Breathing, alone, seemed adequate. I settled my attention into my heart, aware it was resting in God's heart, as happens whenever I pray. The ones who have loved me came to mind, and the ones I have loved. Some of them had come to spend time with me, to bring groceries, to rub my feet. As I thought of my son and my friends, my heart swelled, and tears slipped out of my eyes and puddled in my ears. Despite my fears, I had not been alone without help for long. I had not needed to perform when people came. I was too fatigued to put on a face that pleased. As each person came to visit, I was simply there, with my weak, nonvigilant body and a spread-open heart.

My visitors looked different than usual, not only because I was viewing them from my prone position. Undistracted by my usual agenda of performance and expectation, I was free to notice with heightened awareness the deep timbre of André's voice, how tall he was and with broader shoulders than I remembered, and how he had that looking-toward-the-door, ready-to-rush stance of mine. He brought me a tiny container of essential oil, and I felt loved as Jesus must have when Mary Magdalene sat beside him opening her scent-filled bottles. I noticed Rita's lifted chin, close-lipped smile, tight torso, and swinging hips as she briskly crossed the room to bring me tea. It seemed as if their appearance and everything they said and did arrived moment after moment as another unexpected gift. After they left, the weight of my own head on the pillow felt like a miracle. I thought of the words in my sister's journal near the end of her days: "My being is filled with an inner joy today though the body aches on . . . the love I feel flowing in me is so soothing; it has a healing power that transcends pain." Was I at last beginning to learn the lesson of love my sister had spoken about?

I recovered from Lyme disease within a few weeks. As always when I first get better after an illness, I felt rushes of gratitude as I reclaimed everyday abilities. I delighted in the first moment when I could again lift my head without discomfort, walk across the room with full strength, cook my own meals, and dance. I remember a time years earlier, after a hand injury healed, being thrilled that I could clap again while attending a concert. Sometimes I think the major lesson of illness is to unleash love and appreciation. It's like waking up for the first time and meeting life as a surprise.

In his autobiography, *A Voice at the Borders of Silence*, William Segal, magazine publisher, painter, and spiritual writer, tells of the aftermath of a near-fatal car crash that required fourteen surgeries to remake his severely crushed body. Among other injuries, all his facial bones were broken, and they were separated from his skull. As Segal regained consciousness a few days after the accident, he noticed that his whole body felt "wired together" with tubes everywhere. He could barely breathe or move or see; he could not urinate; and he was in great pain. Segal later wrote about what he decided in that moment: "I said to myself, 'Either I am going to die or I'm not going to die. It's all right. In either case I want to watch to see what goes on.' I dedicated myself entirely to seeing what was happening to my body, to me."

Segal had learned this process of detached, mindful watching from his years of Buddhist discipleship. But it required intentional discipline to maintain this perspective as his body was reconstructed through many surgeries, some successful and some not. He continually recommitted himself to noticing and accepting what happened moment by moment, from the harsh pain after each surgery to the chill he felt when wheeled down a drafty hallway. "My attitude was—accept everything: pain, relief from pain, living, dying." Segal spoke also of finding extraordinary appreciation in the smallest things—the delight in the motion of his wheelchair, the joy in watching the movements of the person cleaning his room.

I remember the same sensations as I lay in my hospital bed shortly after the Lyme disease diagnosis. Doctors were monitoring minor heart problems that caused a temporary worry. Once I began to feel better, every face that appeared in my room seemed like an angel's. Everything I touched seemed like a new toy I'd never played with before. I marveled at my ability to lift my head, to grasp a straw, to notice the eye color of the nurse taking my blood pressure. Gradually, I was reawakening to my body's pleasures and abilities and was flooded with appreciation.

Like Segal, I believe that illness invites transformation. "Serious illness is like a mini-death, at least a foretaste of death," he wrote. "Everything changes." While, as Segal said, "old ways reassert themselves" before long, something underneath is not the same. After a too-long hospital stay, as I awaited the test results and the doctor's release, the keen awareness of my surroundings began to dissipate. The antibiotics had relieved the fever and reduced the aching by then. I was getting impatient to get home. But mostly, after lying around for more than a week, my body was restless and I wanted to *move*. But where is there to go in the heart unit of a hospital? Besides, I was still hooked up to the oxygen tube, though this precaution seemed highly unnecessary since my heart rate had been normal for my whole hospital stay and I was feeling so much better. Still, my body was crying out for some activity, and the only possibility that came to mind was to dance. I had a little space at the foot of my bed, and my bed rail had a small unit attached to it that offered four types of music if I wore a headphone.

What's stopping me, I thought? Hospital rules? "No dancing in the rooms"—unlikely. And even so, maybe it's time I broke a few rules. The risk of looking foolish? My mother's "Don't be so silly" came to mind, but I already looked silly in my hospital dressing gown and besides, who cared? Fear of disturbing some-one? I had no roommate at the moment. Fear of being found out? Well, yes, I realized that someone might walk in on me and be shocked, but I thought, so what? I could just invite them to dance with me, and besides, what fun it would be to see the look on their face! So, nothing was really stopping me. My body wanted to dance, and it was about time I had some fun!

I waited for just the right time. All the morning bath, break-fast, and blood pressure routines were finished. The doctor wouldn't be in for another hour or two. Now's my chance, I thought. Slipping out of bed and into my slippers, I carefully donned the head phones and untangled the cords and tubes linking me to the bed. I peeked out the door to scan the hallway for any personnel likely to intrude, but all were preoccupied. Closing the door, I turned up the rock music. I didn't recognize the tune, but the beat was just right. Yes, it was definitely time to dance.

While we're alive, never a moment passes when our bodies are motionless, silent, or without feeling. They simmer in the juici-ness of life and have a lot to say about what we've been through and what's happening right now, even when hardly anything "works" anymore. They deserve our ongoing reverent attention and appreciation.

Nine years ago, I ran across a newspaper story about former editor in chief of *Elle*, Jean-Dominique Bauby. Though bedrid-den in 1995 after a rare kind of stroke left him with only the capacity to move one eyelid, he learned to blink in patterns so he could communicate. It took him two years, but with the help of an editor who took down each word that Bauby blinked let-ter by letter, he wrote a memoir of his experience, *The Diving Bell and the Butterfly*. He also created a newsletter for others like himself with locked-in syndrome. What most struck me about his tale was not how extraordinarily fertile his wit, courage, and creative passion remained under these conditions, but how the simplest of bodily experiences became amplified for him. He writes of passing a food stand while on a wheelchair ride along a promenade outside the facility where he lived and noticing the dense smell of French fries: "My nostrils quiver with pleasure as they inhale the robust odor." Mostly, though, his ability to enjoy sensory experiences was minimal. He was fed through a tube, unable to savor familiar aromas and tastes. "For pleasure," he wrote, "I have to turn to the vivid memory of tastes and smell, an exhaustible reservoir of sensations." I clipped out the newspaper story about Bauby and have kept it all these years because it reminds me that, no matter our afflictions, we can always find a way to dance, even if all that moves is one eyelid or a pair of quivering nostrils. Our bodies still have moving stories to tell right up until our last breath.

Your Body Odyssey

*M*any people have asked me for ideas on how to learn from their own bodies—how to have their own "body odyssey." Perhaps you'd like to learn how to have greater bodily awareness and freedom yourself. If so, consider trying some of the activities listed below. Each activity is based on a story or idea from one of the book chapters.

There are several ways to make use of these activities. An easy way is to do the activities for a particular chapter right after reading that chapter. Another option is to read the book through and then do the activities, referring to the respective chapters as needed. You can also keep the book handy and pick an activity to try anytime you're ready for a fresh perspective on your life.

If you're unable to perform some of the activities such as standing or lifting your arm, adapt the exercises to fit your abilities. For example, sit or lie down instead of standing, or move a finger in lieu of doing an arm swing.

I encourage you to record your thoughts and feelings in a journal as you do the activities. Or express them in other ways, such as through prayer, meditation, dancing, singing, or making collages. That way you can let your body be involved in the reflecting and recording process as well as in doing the activities themselves. For some of the activities, I make specific suggestions for reflecting on your experience, but I encourage you to let your own creative impulses guide you.

In general, these activities are intended to be pleasurable opportunities for you to learn and grow. If you suspect any of them may arouse emotions too difficult for you to handle alone, please seek the guidance of a therapist or other professional before doing it.

Here are some tips that will help you get the most out of these activities:

- Do the activities slowly, with mindful attention.
- Observe your reactions much the way you'd watch a new baby, delighting in every gesture and grimace.
- Watch and listen with your "inside" eyes, ears, and other sensations. Be patient with yourself as you attempt this new way of observing your experience.
- Do the exercises as experiments and enjoy any discoveries you make, even it they are small.
- Look for more ways you can tune in to your body's communication during day-to-day activities. Consider further study of body awareness disciplines such as the Feldenkrais Method.

Here is an introductory exercise* to help you get started with feeling the aliveness within your body:

Stand with your eyes closed. Feel yourself living inside each area of your body. Do this slowly, taking time to breathe freely as you notice your experience in each area. Begin by feeling yourself living inside your feet, then inside your ankles, calves, knees, thighs, pelvis, belly, midsection, chest, shoulders, upper arms, elbows, lower arms, wrists, hands, neck, and head. Feel yourself inside your whole body. Staying inside your body, feel yourself

* Adapted from the Subtle Self work of Judith Blackstone (see "Other Helpful Resources," p. 221).

living within the space around you. Open your eyes. Move into the space around you, staying inside your whole body.

Enjoy your body odyssey!

Chapter One: When Terror Wants to Have Its Say

(A) Bring to mind an experience that felt physically threatening—perhaps a close call to a fall or car accident, or a threat by another person. How did your body feel during the event? In the days following? See if you can re-experience that feeling now. Spend a few minutes observing the feeling without trying to change it. Simply let the feeling be there and notice if it changes as you observe it.

(B) Think back to a situation where you felt conflicting emotions. Perhaps you were scared of someone but also felt a desire to help this person. You may have experienced this type of inner conflict when meeting a homeless beggar. Put yourself back in this situation, re-experiencing as fully as possible the thoughts and feelings you had at the time. Then, observe how your body reacts when you turn your attention to each of these various thoughts and feelings. For example, notice how "scared" feels in your body. Then, notice how "desire to help" feels. The differences may be very subtle. If you have trouble noticing them at first, try looking for slight changes in your facial expression and tummy tension.

Chapter Two: From Cover to Uncover

(A) The next time you're with other members of your family, notice how they walk, sit, gesture. When they speak, notice the volume, tone, and pitch of their voices. Compare your own movement and vocal qualities with theirs. Reflect on how the qualities you have picked up from your family have shaped your life.

(B) People may sometimes comment on your getting old, saying things like, "What can you expect at your age?" or "You're not as young as you used to be, you know." If they do, how do you react? Notice the thoughts that come to mind about your body. Pay attention to your physical reactions, such as putting your hand somewhere on your body that you think feels or looks "old." What are these reactions based on?

(C) Stand comfortably on both feet. Become attentive to how you're standing. Without changing anything, notice if your weight is more on one foot than the other. If you're unable to stand, notice as you're sitting or lying if your weight is more on one side of your body than another. By simple acts of observing your body like this, you can begin to discover the desires and wisdom it holds.

Chapter Three: Turning 50

(A) What were some of the rules you learned as a child regarding your body? What "rules" have you learned about how you should act as you get older? Complete this sentence: "If I made the rules . . ."

(B) Arrange a time to be at home alone. Put on music that is sensual and soulful. Let yourself dance without restraint.

(C) Imagine a celebration of your decade birthday that would honor your body's deepest longings. What would you do? Feel the thrill of white-water rafting? Rock children on your lap? Have a sing-along in the moonlight by an echo-producing canyon? Draw, paint, or make up a song about this experience. Or create the actual celebration to match your desires.

Chapter Four: The Body as Metaphor and Mirror

(A) Scan your body until you find an area of pain or discomfort. Name that area (such as "my neck tension") and complete the sentence: "Sometimes (my painful area) is like . . ." ten or more times. Choose one of your responses and write a playful poem or story based upon it.

(B) Move your right arm around in a big circle. Do the same with your left arm. Notice which arm does the motion more easily. Do the motion again with that arm, restricting the movement to match the way the other arm is restricted. Then do the motion again with both arms and notice any differences in your freedom of movement.

Chapter Five: No Brakes

(A) Visit an art gallery. Notice your body's response as you view the exhibits. If some works make you tense, where does the tension arise in your body? If some works please you, notice whether you stand taller, smile, feel a softness in your belly, or have other responses. If any of the artworks remind you of something in your own life, does that memory rest in your jaw, heart, lungs, pelvis?

(B) Think of an old friend or partner you no longer see. Imagine suddenly running into that person. How does your body respond? Does this response suggest any unfinished business you still have with this person? If so, consider writing, "What I still want to say to [person] is . . ." Listen to your body as you write.

Chapter Six: Carrying Weights

(A) Play an instrument if you have one, and while playing, notice what is happening in your body. What moves? Is there tension or ease in the movement? Is any part of your body moving other than the ones needed to play the instrument? What is prompting those movements? Experiment with changing the tension level and the movements as you play. Notice how these changes affect the quality of the music and of your overall experience.

(B) Take note of the music-related objects you have in your home—music instruments, CD player, CDs, songbooks. Pick up one of them. As you hold it, recall any people or experiences associated with it. Observe your body reactions as you do this.

(C) Sit quietly, away from noise as much as possible. Listen inwardly for a sound, a melody, a music all your own. Let this listening go beyond your ears to your whole body, in the same way as your whole body takes in the experience of hearing a drumbeat. Take your time. If no sound becomes apparent, make one up. Let it be heard, even if it's just a tiny hum. Let it get bigger and then smaller. Vary the tonal quality, the pace. Put words to it, if you like. Later, consider sharing it with someone who loves you.

Chapter Seven: Slow Down the Hurry Up

(A) Write for five minutes, beginning with "My mother always said . . ." Then reflect on how these parental messages took hold in your body. For example, how do they affect the speed with which you move, the way you carry your shoulders, the amount of food you eat?

(B) Consider taking a period of sabbath—a day, a week, a year. Find a place to go where you can be undistracted by your usual activities. Still your mind as much as possible and tune in to your body's wishes and wisdom.

Chapter Eight: The Silent Sanctuaries of Shame

(A) Make a list of religious rituals and practices from your childhood, such as kneeling, bowing, fasting, and lighting candles. Choose one and journal about what it meant to you then and how it has shaped your choices over the years. You can do the same with each of the items on your list.

(B) Choose one of the items on the above list that was a personal religious practice for you. Do the activity mindfully, noticing all the movements and sensations associated with it. Consider whether you wish to continue doing this activity on a regular basis, adapt it to make it more suitable to your current situation, or simply honor it as a part of shaping who you are.

(C) When someone criticizes you or questions your views, pay attention to what happens in your body. Do you turn red, avert your eyes, feel tension in your belly? Do your jaw muscles firm up? Does your heart speed up? Do your fists start to tighten into balls? What is the story behind these responses?

Chapter Nine: Panic

(A) Try this exercise the next time you are feeling anxious. Step back from your anxiety as best you can and observe the reactions of your body and mind one by one. Describe aloud what you're noticing or write it down: "My heart is beating faster. My face is hot. I'm having trouble breathing. I feel a zinging sensation in my brain." Describe your thinking: "I'm having thoughts about wanting to calm down and get this under control." Your purpose is not to change anything that is happening. In fact, avoid trying to change anything. That may only increase your anxiety. Simply *notice* what is happening, as a compassionate but detached observer would. You cannot do this exercise wrong. Its only purpose is to invite greater awareness. Over time, this attentive observing of your experience may diminish your anxiety or panic.

(B) When you feel anxious, think of a song that is soothing for you and sing or hum it to yourself. If other people are around who might be willing to sing to you in a loving way, consider asking them to do so.

Chapter Ten: *Say It with Eggs*

(A) Remember a time when you felt angry. What were your thoughts about these angry feelings? Did you savor your righteous stance? Did you feel guilty? Did you try to push the anger away? Depending in part on your thoughts, your body may have become tense, experienced a burst of energy, or had other responses. The next time you feel angry, be aware of these sensations and movements in your body. Notice the thoughts related to them. Watch them come and go without judging or changing them. Jot down what you observe. Notice how this mindful attention affects your experience of anger.

(B) Take a carton of eggs into the woods. Go alone or invite a friend or two to join you. Toss eggs at a tree, one by one. As you do, freely and loudly express your upsetting feelings. Make this exercise serious or fun—your choice! Afterward, pay attention to whether you have a greater range of emotional expression available to you in your day-to-day life.

(C) If you could sing your own personal freedom song, what would it be? Start exploring by humming or mouthing "ohhh" or "hey" or "sss." From this initial sound let words form. Don't censor yourself. You can also start with words such as "yes," "no," "I want," or "I am," and add to them as you are moved to do so. If you have trouble getting started with this activity, begin by taking a few deep breaths. On the third or fourth exhalation, let a sound—any sound—spill out in full force. As your sound develops, let it expand into a song. Feel free to add movements that illustrate the song or give it greater impulse. It's best, of course, to do this activity where your full volume can be expressed without disturbing others—in your car, a country setting, or at home alone.

Chapter Eleven: Transcendental Bodies

(A) Walk a labyrinth. If no labyrinth is available, then find an open space—preferably outdoors—and walk in a spiral pattern, following at first a large circular path that gradually spirals inward to a point at the center; then follow the same path back out to your starting point. Walk slowly and mindfully, touching the ground with each step as if doing so were a brand-new experience. Drop your thoughts like pebbles along the way. Let your attention be on your walking. Do a before-and-after check on how your body feels. Notice how this walk influences the rest of your day.

(B) Take a walk in nature or around your neighborhood and be on the lookout for objects such as feathers, leaves, and flower petals that delight your senses and lift your spirits. Gather these objects and place them in a special place at home, creating a shrine to help you remember what your body enjoys. Add sacred objects such as candles or statues. Whenever you handle the objects at your shrine, notice their shape, texture, weight, color, firmness, aroma, sound, and other qualities. Use these objects to help you create meaningful spiritual rituals.

(C) Create a story doll that reflects your religious history. Use a wine carafe or a bottle you like as a base. If possible, choose a container that has some resemblance in size and shape to your own body. Cover it with cloth or craft materials. Use a foam or cloth ball to make the doll's head. Adorn the doll with items representing your faith experience. Use your imagination as you did when you were a child. Lace draped over the head could represent a communion veil—or a starry crown, the Virgin Mary. Include jewelry using symbols such as feathers or crosses from your faith tradition. Attach to the doll's clothing photos from important moments such as a bar or bat mitzvah. When the doll is finished, show it to your children, grandchildren, or children in your faith community and tell them the story of your doll. Write a prayer or artist's statement to display with it.

Chapter Twelve: Hangin' Out

(A) Notice an area of your body that is often tense. Give yourself at least ten minutes to tend to this area. During this time, regard the tense area with high interest. Do not try to relax or relieve it. Rather, let the tense area have its say and listen with great care. Pay attention to exactly where the tension is within the particular area of discomfort. How large is it? What shape? Is the tension static or moving around? Which direction is the pull, if there is one? Let compassion for this area of your body arise in your heart. Invite the tension to make itself even more apparent. Does it get bigger? Move? Intensify? Welcome whatever is happening and follow it with your attention. Let your body move according to whatever impulses arise. Stay interested and allow your body to tell its story in its own way. Notice memories, images, or emotions that appear. You may begin to get insights about your area of tension. Observe how your body, thoughts, and feelings change as you stay welcoming and observant. Stay with this process until it feels complete in some way for you. Journal about your experience. If you have difficulty with the process, find a bodyworker or therapist with experience in somatic learning or therapy who can help you.

Chapter Thirteen: Born to Be Wild

(A) Close your eyes, quiet your mind, and relax. Find a scar on your body. In your imagination, slowly explore, caress, and cherish the scar. Remember the story of how it came to you. Give it a separate identity, a name, a voice. Place your pen in the hands of your scar. Invite your scar to write a letter addressed to you in which your scar tells you about all the wisdom it represents: wisdom about pain and healing, injury and recovery, vulnerability and perseverance, risk and adventure, fracture and renewal, wounds and wholeness. Open your eyes and begin writing.

(B) Remember a time when you were physically adventurous, perhaps as a child. Recall the feelings and sensations you had— the shakiness, antsy feeling, or rush of energy. Maybe you had stomach butterflies or a headache before you started the activity. Perhaps you got very tired, sore, or even injured. What "story" did you create about yourself and about life as a result of this adventure? How has that story affected your ability to take risks, physical and otherwise?

(C) Notice some place you're *holding* in your body—a tight muscle, a bending or contraction. Holding is a means of protecting yourself. Keep on holding. Tighten the holding until you feel sufficiently protected. Become aware of what you're protecting yourself from. Notice any fear, anger, or other feelings contained in that holding. Notice any memories that come to mind. Notice any thoughts that you try to dismiss, perhaps in an attempt to protect yourself. Pay attention to what's happening to your holding as you observe your thoughts and feelings. Has it shifted in any way? Notice if there is any way to loosen the feeling of holding and still feel safe.

Chapter Fourteen: Writing from the Body

(A) If you write in a journal, where do you sit to do so? In what posture? Take note of your surroundings—lighting, furnishings, textures, colors, sounds. Change some or all of these aspects of your journaling experience for a few days. For example, sit in a different chair, write with your mouth open, or play background music that's unusual for you. Notice how this change affects the way you write.

(B) Look around your home for something old and precious to you. Spend a few minutes enjoying this item with your senses. Look at it. Feel its size, weight, texture, and temperature. Explore any sounds it makes when you handle it. Write a few paragraphs about it, beginning with, "This reminds me of . . ."

(C) Writing comes alive when it contains sentient details. Recall a recent experience and remember how you used your senses to take it in. Try to recall and re-experience these sensory activities as vividly as you can, as if the event were happening in this moment. Then write a description of the experience. Include as much sensory detail as possible.

Chapter Fifteen: Bear the Body, Bare the Soul . . . And Let the Dancing Begin

(A) Remember what it was like to be carried as a child? Have you ever been carried by anyone since you've been an adult? Remember the feeling of surrendering and letting your weight drop, the feeling of support as caring hands and arms held you. Or perhaps you recall your body becoming tense or pained if you were carried against your will. How do these memories affect your ability now to seek and accept support from others— emotionally and physically? Jot down your thoughts.

(B) Have you ever had a massage where you felt like you were being held and nurtured by the person giving the massage? Consider gathering a few close, trusted friends together for the purpose of giving each other mutual foot rubs, shoulder massages, or scalp massages. Sing or hum to each other, like a mother might do when comforting a sick child.

(C) Are you always the one who carries others? Is the weight of the world on your shoulders? Notice if your body has taken any particular shape or tension as a result. Maybe you have worry lines, stooped shoulders, or excessive weight. Imagine yourself as a child being carried securely by someone you trust deeply. Observe how your body responds to this image.

(D) At this moment, pay attention to the urges simmering within your body. Are you feeling fierce, slinky, skittery, chirpy, slothful? Imagine yourself as an animal that reflects what your body is feeling. Let yourself move and make noises like that animal would. Exaggerate these movements and noises. Enjoy feeling the spirit of this animal as you express it. Journal about any discoveries you make.

Chapter Sixteen: *The Language of the Body Is Spoken Here*

(A) Bring your attention to your face. Notice any tension there. Welcome this tension. Gradually exaggerate it. Keep exaggerating it, until that tension is fully expressed. Let your neck, shoulders, and the rest of the body follow along if they want to. How familiar is this tension? What is it saying? What story, experience, or image does it brings to mind? How does it feel to honor the experience of your face in this way?

(B) Practice saying "no" in front of a mirror. Say it in various ways—fearfully, brazenly, comically, in a teasing way, respectfully. Vary the volume. As you say each no, be aware of your posture, movements, facial expression, and feeling of energy. Have fun with this exercise. Use it as a warm-up for saying a no you need to say.

(C) Observe yourself at a meeting, class, or other long-sitting event. What is your body experiencing? How is this experience affecting your ability to learn, enjoy, and participate?

(D) Remember the last time you greatly enjoyed learning something. Try to recall and re-experience how your body participated in the learning. Look for ways to draw upon this experience to help you learn in other situations.

Chapter Seventeen: Dances of the Heart

(A) Put on some music and do a mirroring exercise with a friend. Take turns mirroring the movements of each other without talking. Pay attention to how it feels to have your moves noticed and adopted by another. As you follow your partner's moves, have fun trying out someone else's way of moving. Talk about your discoveries with your partner.

(B) The next time you get together with a group of friends, bring along a ball, lively music, and a playful spirit. Invite everyone to break the usual routine and play catch, dance, play mime games, or engage in other physical activities. Notice your mood and energy level afterward.

Chapter Eighteen: Bodies in Pain

(A) Make a list of your chronic body ailments. Choose one of them. Give it a name and a personality. (One friend of mine called her tumor Penelope.) Write, dance, act out, or tell the story of your ailment from the point of view of the personality you chose. If you can share this expression with a circle of the caring people in your life, all the better.

(B) Write a letter to your illness, expressing your fears, concerns, and questions about it. Write a letter back to yourself, letting the wisdom of the illness reply.

(C) When you feel pain or other discomfort, consider what would most help your body feel better at that moment. If that help is not available, close your eyes and imagine someone giving your body exactly what it wants in a very nurturing way. Make the image as strong as possible, much like an athlete does when mentally practicing for a game or race. Feel every detail of the aid coming your way and notice how your body is responding.

(D) Pay attention to what feels healthy in your body. Spend an extended period of time noticing and appreciating everything that works—from your eyelids blinking to your skin protecting you. Thank your body for being your home and for doing its best to keep you comfortable and healthy.

Bibliography

Bauby, Jean-Dominique. *The Diving Bell and the Butterfly*. New York: Albert A. Knopf, 1997.

Bemis, Judith, and Barrada, Amr. *Embracing the Fear: Learning to Manage Anxiety and Panic Attacks*. Center City, MN: Hazelden, 1994.

Budd, Matthew, and Rothstein, Larry. *You Are What You Say*. New York: Three Rivers Press, 2000.

Childre, Doc, and Martin, Howard. *The HeartMath Solution*. New York: HarperSanFrancisco, 1999.

Damasio, Antonio. *The Feeling of What Happens*. San Diego: Harcourt, 1999.

Fillmore, Myrtle. *Myrtle Fillmore's Healing Letters*. Reader: Rosemary Fillmore Rhea. Unity Village, MO: Unity, 1988.

Hanh, Thich Nhat. *Touching Peace: Practicing the Art of Mindful Living*. Berkeley: Parallax Press, 1992.

Hillman, James. *The Force of Charcter and the Lasting Life*. New York: Random House, 1999.

Keen, Sam. *Learning to Fly*. New York: Broadway Books, 1999.

Lowe, Bia. *Wild Ride*. San Francisco: HarperCollins, 1996.

Montagu, Ashley. *Growing Young*. Westport, CT: Bergin & Garvcy, 1989.

Moore, Thomas. *Care of the Soul*. New York: HarperPerennial, 1992.

Moore, Thomas. *Care of the Soul*. Reader: Peter Thomas. HarperCollins Publishers, 1992.

Paley, Grace. "Travelling." *New Yorker* 8 Sept. 1997.

Rabbit-Proof Fence. Dir. Phillip Noyce. Perf. Evelyn Sampi, Tianna Sansbury, Laura Monaghan, David Gulpilil, Kenneth Branagh, and Myarn Lawford. Miramax, 2002.

Riedman, Sister Patricia Ann, P.B.M. Untitled speech. Maryvale, Valley City, ND. 1 Jan. 1983.

Sanders, Scott Russell. "Witnessing to a Shared World." *A View from the Loft,* Winter, 1997: 13+.

Schank, Roger C. *Tell Me a Story: Narrative and Intelligence.* Evanston, IL: Northwestern University, 1990.

Segal, William. *A Voice at the Borders of Silence: The Autobiography of William Segal.* Woodstock, NY: Overlook Press, 2003.

Snyder, Gary. *The Practice of the Wild.* New York: North Point Press, 1990.

Stroh, Sister Kevin, P.B.M. "Dear Sisters." *Marynotes* 18.2 (1983): 1–2.

Taylor, Daniel. *The Healing Power of Stories.* New York: Doubleday, 1996. (Republished as *Tell Me a Story: The Life-Shaping Power of Our Stories.* St. Paul, MN: Bog Walk Press, 2001.)

Wuthrow, Robert. *Creative Spirituality: The Way of the Artist.* Berkeley: University of California Press, 2001.

Other Helpful Resources

www.congoldman.org Describes the work of Connie Goldman, author of *The Aging Spirit,* radio producer, and longtime spokesperson for vital aging.

www.creativeaging.org The National Center for Creative Aging Web site, featuring resources on creative aging, including contact information for artists throughout the nation who engage older adults in the arts.

www.feldenkrais.com The Feldenkrais Educational Foundation of America provides information about the Feldenkrais Method and how to find local practitioners.

www.essential-motion.com Features information about Karen Roeper's work on personal transformation through movement.

www.groupmotion.org Gives information about the Philadelphia-based Group Motion Dance Company, which offers weekly improvisational dance opportunities as well as weeklong retreats around the nation for the public.

www.heartmath.org and www.heartmath.com Describes the HeartMath Institute's scientific studies and other resources that shed light on the power of the heart and show how to access it for less stress and better health.

www.hakomiinstitute.com Offers information on Hakomi mind/body therapy and provides a directory of practitioners.

www.inventuregroup.com Highlights the work of Richard Leider, author of *Claiming Your Place at the Fire: Living the Second Half of Your Life on Purpose,* helping people live their purpose.

www.laviniaplonka.com Describes the body awareness work of Feldenkrais teacher Lavinia Plonka and has information about her book *What Are You Afraid Of?*

www.pbsp.com Provides information on Pesso Boyden System Psychomotor, a comprehensive therapeutic approach to trauma healing that involves creating alternate virtual memories in the mind and body.

www.realizationcenter.com Offers information on the Subtle Self work of Judith Blackstone, which teaches attunement to fundamental consciousness through the body.

www.van.umn.edu Describes the work of the Vital Aging Network in Minnesota and offers many other resources on aging.

Knaster, Mirka. *Discover the Body's Wisdom.* New York: Bantam, 1996. Provides an excellent introductory overview of more than fifty mind-body practices.

Osho, *Body Mind Balancing.* New York: St. Martin's Griffin,

2003. Offers kindly admonitions and practical ideas from a respected spiritual teacher about befriending our bodies.

Plonka, Lavinia. *What Are You Afraid of? A Body/Mind Guide to Courageous Living.* New York: Tarcher/Penguin, 2004. Provides practical exercises to locate and heal the patterns of fear we carry in our bodies.

Scarf, Maggie. *Secrets, Lies, Betrayals.* New York: Random House, 2004. Provides a neurobiological understanding of how our bodies store memories of trauma and how those memories can be accessed so that healing can take place.

Pat Samples, M.A., M.F.A., is a writer, international speaker, and transformational educator. She is the author of six books in addition to *Body Odyssey*, including *Daily Comforts for Caregivers*, and has written widely on health, aging, and human behavior. She speaks and gives workshops on conscious aging, body wisdom, caregiving, creative living, and other personal development topics. Samples is a past editor of *The Phoenix*, a wellness monthly, and the former director of an arts education center. She has master's degrees in creative writing and human development, and she teaches writing courses for local universities.

In her writing, speaking, and teaching, Samples draws on her experience working and volunteering in health care, social services, ministry, and the arts. She helps people recognize and draw upon their own wisdom, including the wisdom of their body, to reveal, celebrate, and revise the stories they live by. More than 300 organizations and events have hosted her talks and workshops, including state and national conferences on aging and caregiving, Area Agencies on Aging, wellness organizations and expos, writing and creativity conferences, Alzheimer's Associations, Catholic Charities, Lutheran Social Service, senior centers and residences, social work and nursing organizations, churches and ministry groups, women's organizations, and many more.

Samples lives in a Minneapolis suburb, where the egrets in the pond behind her home teach her of beauty and stillness and the weeping willows remind her to bend with the wind.

For more information about Pat Samples and her speaking schedule, visit:

www.agingandcaregiving.com

For information, tips, and other resources regarding the body's creativity and wisdom, visit her Body Odyssey Web site:

www.bodyodyssey.biz

To order additional copies of *Body Odyssey*

Web: www.itascabooks.com

Phone: 1-800-901-3480

Fax: Copy and fill out the form below with credit card information. Fax to 763-398-0198.

Mail: Copy and fill out the form below. Mail with check or credit card information to:

Syren Book Company
5120 Cedar Lake Road
Minneapolis, MN 55416

Order Form

Copies	Title / Author	Price	Totals
	***Body Odyssey* / Pat Samples**	$15.95	$
		Subtotal	$
		7% sales tax (MN only)	$
		Shipping and handling, first copy	$ 4.00
		Shipping and handling, ___ add'l copies @$1.00 ea.	$
		TOTAL TO REMIT	$

Payment Information:

___ Check enclosed   ___ Visa/MasterCard
Card number: Expiration date:
Name on card:
Billing address:
City: State: Zip:
Signature :   Date:

Shipping Information:

___ Same as billing address   ___ Other (enter below)
Name:
Address:
City: State: Zip: